Martin Bates is the pseudonym of an established British writer with a personal interest in high blood pressure. Diagnosed hypertensive in 1965, he has tried most of the drug types he describes and has been helped to a low and stable blood pressure by the kind of information his book contains.

High Blood Pressure

How to Live With It
How to Lower It

MARTIN BATES

A SPECTRUM BOOK

Prentice-Hall, Inc. Englewood Cliffs, New Jersey 07632

Library of Congress Cataloging in Publication Data

Bates, Martin.
High blood pressure.

"A Spectrum Book."
Rev. ed. of: Living with high blood pressure. 1980.
Bibliography: p.
Includes index.
1. Hypertension—Prevention. 2. Hypertension—Treatment. I. Title.
RC685.H8B33 1982 616.1'32 81-22724
AACR2

ISBN 0-13-387381-1

ISBN 0-13-387373-0 {PBK.}

This Spectrum Book is available to businesses and organizations at a special discount when ordered in large quantities. For information, contact Prentice-Hall, Inc., General Publishing Division, Special Sales, Englewood Cliffs, N. J. 07632.

A SPECTRUM BOOK

10 9 8 7 6 5 4 3 2 1

Printed in the United States of America

Prentice-Hall International, Inc., *London*
Prentice-Hall of Australia Pty. Limited, *Sydney*
Prentice-Hall of Canada, Ltd., *Toronto*
Prentice-Hall of India Private Limited, *New Delhi*
Prentice-Hall of Japan, Inc., *Tokyo*
Prentice-Hall of Southeast Asia Pte. Ltd., *Singapore*
Whitehall Books Limited, *Wellington, New Zealand*

Contents

Acknowledgments

For their helpful response to his inquiries the author is indebted to the British Medical Association, Roche Products Limited, the staffs of Messrs H.K. Lewis, the London Library and the British Library, also to all members of the medical profession who have assisted him.

1

The Quiet Problem

In an age of easy communication, high blood pressure remains a curiously obscure phenomenon. The very term doctors use to refer to it—*hypertension,* which means quite simply high blood pressure—is a kind of disguise against recognition. Many people know nothing of it; more misjudge the problems.

This is surprising and regrettable.

Surprising, because hypertension is the most common of the chronic health conditions known to Western medicine. It has been estimated that 24 million people in the United States are hypertensive. In England, more than five in every 100 adults are reckoned to need treatment, and other countries face the same exigency.

Almost certainly everybody in a modern Western environment knows someone at work, or socially, with hypertension.

Surprising, then, that the problem is not better understood. And regrettable, because lack of public information contributes to indifference not only among people at large but even among those under treatment. A major problem cited by doctors is the failure of hypertensive patients to comply seriously with the treatment prescribed for them. No more than a minority of the hypertensives in Europe and the United States, it is calculated, have their condition under adequate control, despite the availability of easy detection and simple treatment in pill form.

Why should this be? Hypertension is simply diagnosed. Treatment that lowers the blood pressure is effective in the vast majority of cases, and lower pressure greatly reduces health risks. Why should relatively little have been heard by the public about hypertension at a time when newspapers, television, billboards, and doctors' waiting-rooms regularly inform the world about health problems and preventive measures of many kinds?

For a long while, unsure as to the cause of the condition and lacking means of controlling it, the medical profession was sensibly chary of pronouncements on the subject. Also, aware of the possibility of aggravating the condition by worrying those affected, doctors tended to play down the seriousness of high blood presure to their patients. But so encouraging has been the record of new drug treatments in recent years that today the facts themselves are more comforting than the old platitudes.

In the past decade an increasing number of doctors has advocated mass screening for hypertension. In Britain, many members of the medical profession take the view that planned diagnosis could and should be organized under the National Health Service to discover and treat the unknown hypertensives in the community. In the United States, a national committee formed to detect and treat high blood pressure recommends both screening and a program of public education. Hypertension, it is recognized, does not advertise itself. Indeed, often—almost always, some doctors would say—it is without warning symptoms. Even those persons with extremely high blood pressure may neither feel nor appear ill. Nor, where it applies, does the somewhat nebulous "under the weather" sensation that sometimes accompanies the condition cause much alarm.

Cut your hand, it has been said, and someone will rush you to a hospital for a stitch, but describe what you feel—if anything—with hypertension and the same person will wink and say you must have enjoyed yourself the night before. Add to the inconspicuous nature of the condition the fact that a great many known hypertensives cope resourcefully without fuss, and the covertness of the problem becomes easier to understand.

Typical of many with a blood pressure problem and a tough job is a dynamic woman in her mid-forties who specializes in dealing with problem children and their misdemeanors at a large school. She thrives on it. In her spare time, apart from horseback riding with her husband and daughter and a hectic program of entertaining, she has organized the women of her local community into a mutual-aid catering group to cut the expenses of weddings and other functions. She has lived with hypertension for many years, but seldom mentions it. She respects it and the rules of medication—and pitches into life.

An architect, diagnosed hypertensive thirteen years ago, told me recently: "I'm fifty-three now. I still work hard, though more sensibly than I did before the treatment. I've learned when to stop. At first the pressure-lowering drugs made life unusual, but you soon adjust. Today, I might never have had problems, the way I feel." Living with hypertension has not diminished his zest for a taxing, creative business with demanding details. He looks healthy, suntanned, and leanly fit.

Neither of these people advocates disregarding the dangers of hypertension. Acquainted with the facts, they are careful to abide by the advice of their doctors concerning medicine, reducing weight, cutting down on alcohol, not smoking, and so on. They have tackled treatment thoroughly, regardless of initial inconvenience. It is not something they dwell on.

Like so many hypertensives, who are often intelligent individuals of drive and energy, they thrust forward rather than look back. Their standpoint is enlightenment, not ignorance. Countless men and women pursue successful careers while controlling hypertensive tendencies; countless more would live naturally, despite high blood pressure, into active old age.

Much anxiety is unnecessary. In the vast majority of cases, high blood pressure is a sign, not an illness—a sign that preventive steps may be advisable. For if neglected, the risk of its becoming an illness is greater than when controlled. So, say many doctors, public education is desirable both in the cause of promoting treatment and in getting the most from it.

Modern medication has worked wonders for the hypertensive, but getting full value demands adjustments of mind and, in the early stages, perseverance with an uncustomary regimen. There is no doubt that the scope for sensible self-help in the process is considerable.

A balanced attitude is invaluable. Since the facts about the subject are today so reassuring, it is deplorable that people should remain worried through ignorance. Ignorance is no position from which to face any problem, especially one that may feed on the fear and awe it generates.

In the following pages it is my purpose first, to replace fear with understanding; second, to place the subject simply and informatively in perspective; and, third, to pass on from fellow hypertensives, as well as doctors, some useful hints on living with high blood pressure.

2

About Blood Pressure

What is blood pressure? To understand that, it is necessary to have an idea of how the blood circulates in the body—something mankind took a long time to find out.

Although the ancient Greeks recognized the veins as blood channels, their views on the arteries were curious. Herophilus, founder of the Alexandrian school of medicine and the first anatomist to compare the human body with that of other creatures, taught that the arteries carried air or "spirit."

Most of the Greek doctors appear to have thought that the veins, not the arteries, carried blood from heart to members. Aristotle, for instance, believed that blood was produced in the liver, moved to the heart, and thence by the veins through the body.

Some centuries later, when Galen, the innovator of diagnosis by the pulse, discovered blood in the arteries, he too thought they carried "spirit." His views persisted until the sixteenth century. At that time—the age of Luther and the Spanish Armada—doctors believed that the movements of blood in the body were irregular in direction and that, though generally sluggish, they were of varying speeds.

They also believed that there were two kinds of blood in a body—one in the veins, flowing by the right chamber or ventricle of the heart, and the other in the arteries, flowing by the left ventricle. That the heart actually provided the motor power to move the blood was unknown to them.

It was not until the seventeenth century, after a long series of dissections and observations, including that of the conveniently transparent shrimp, that the English physician William Harvey published in fifty-two brilliant pages his great discovery of the circulation of the blood. Among other things, Harvey showed:

That the mover of the blood is the heart.

That the ventricles of the heart pump the blood into the arteries.

That the pulse is produced by the arteries being filled with blood.

That there is complete circulation of the blood by arteries and veins.

That the blood in all parts of the body is the same blood.

That the blood flows in a constant and steady stream.

Today it is known that the movement through the various vessel circuits is so rapid that it normally takes less than a minute for a given particle of blood to pass from the heart and return to it. Briefly, its progress is as follows: From the heart, it passes by a single tube, the *aorta* or trunk artery. This divides and redivides into progressively smaller arteries until, from the smallest, the blood passes into tiny vessels called *capillaries.* It is through the fine walls of the capillaries that the blood supplies the various regions of the body with nourishment and oxygen (collected on its journey from the intestine and the lungs), gathering at the same time waste products for disposal by the kidneys and other channels.

Having traveled from the heart to the capillaries, the blood returns by a reverse of the branching process. The tiny vessels join to form somewhat larger ones, which in turn merge in bigger tubes, *veins,* the blood at last regaining the heart through two large veins.

The prime mover of the blood on this journey is the rhythmic pumping action the heart achieves by means of the thick muscular walls that bound its cavities. By so pumping, the heart creates sufficient pressure in the arteries to impel the blood on its round trip. Understandably, since the pressure diminishes the farther the blood proceeds, the force is greater in the arteries than in the veins.

MEASUREMENT OF BLOOD PRESSURE

Harvey's discovery of the circulation of the blood implied a pressure in the system, but its measurement was still far off. In the eighteenth century, an inquisitive British clergyman, Stephen Hales, became the first person to measure blood pressure directly by observing the height to which blood spurted from the artery of a horse. For more than a hundred years the only methods of measurement were similarly direct and confined to use on animals.

By 1850 the mercury pressure gauge had been introduced as the result of work by, among others, Karl Ludwig, the German physiologist. Doctors began to consider the possibility of measuring arterial pulsation externally. The principle they adopted was ingenious—measure the counter-pressure necessary to obliterate the pulsations in a peripheral artery (the large one in the arm was convenient) and use this as an index of blood pressure. It remained to design an instrument.

First attempts were clumsy and unreliable. In 1876 a Viennese physician named Von Basch designed an apparatus that employed a diaphragm stretched over a glass funnel to compress the artery. A decade later, a more compact version replaced the diaphragm and funnel with a rubber bulb, one finger pressing this on the artery while another sought the point at which the pulse was obliterated. As its inventor admitted, a frequent source of error was the ease with which the pulse of the doctor's finger could be mistaken for that of the patient.

The forerunner of the familiar instrument used today, the sphygmomanometer, was designed by a professor of medicine at the University of Padua and first described in a paper he published in 1896. Professor Riva-Rocci's apparatus was comprised of three parts: a cuff applied to the upper arm, an inflating bulb, and a mercury gauge or manometer. Marketed the same year by the Zambelli Company of Turin, it had a somewhat shorter mercury column than that in present use, and its cuff was narrower. At the beginning of this century it was pointed out that the 4.5-cm cuff of the original gave unduly high readings and the 12-cm cuff of today was put in its place. Otherwise, the apparatus has not changed significantly.

Two measurements of blood pressure are taken, the doctor timing the heart action by using a stethoscope on a pulse; a high, which occurs during the contraction of the heart, and is known as the *systolic,* and a low, which occurs during the relaxation of the heart, and is known as the *diastolic.*

For convenience, the pressures are equated in millimetres to the pressure exerted by the column of mercury. A typical reading is, say, a systolic pressure of 120 mm of mercury with a diastolic pressure of 80 mm—expressed concisely as 120/80 mm.

It is not possible, though the phrase is sometimes heard, to define "normal blood pressure" with any meaning because there are variations, not only among groups and individuals, but in the same person at different times. For instance, blood pressure is lower in childhood than in adulthood. The most rapid rise occurs between birth and the mid-teens, young adulthood being a period of little change until, from about the age of thirty-five to forty, pressure rises slowly to around the age of sixty-five, after which there is not much alteration.

In childhood, boys and girls have the same blood pressure values, but as they grow up females have a rather lower blood pressure on average than males until the menopause, after which the position is reversed. From the age of sixty, the average pressure in women is significantly higher than that in men—an effect, it appears, of selection. Women tolerate high pressures much better than men and live longer as a result.

Temporary variations in blood pressure are caused, of course, by physical and emotional activity. Everyone knows that the heart pounds after a rush to catch a train or bus—or, indeed, after athletic endeavor of other kinds. Pressure may rise as a consequence of anger, fear, guilt, or excitement of different types. The so-called "lie detector" picks up emotional reaction to a crucial challenge by recording the change in blood pressure. Sexual arousal and performance involve increased blood pressure—a prerequisite of male potency.

Although such fluctuations occur in individuals, mean levels, and the rates at which they increase with age, vary markedly in the community.

Long-term observation of groups of men disclosed that about a third had little increase in blood pressure over a thirty-year period. Of the rest, most had a slow rise in pressure, a small number showing a more rapid rise. Those with initially low or average pressures displayed lower rates of increase during the period than those who started with higher blood pressures.

With a view to preventive treatment, it would clearly be helpful if those persons likely to develop the higher pressures in later life could be identified while still young. Such people often have passing phases of high pressure before the feature becomes persistent.

Unfortunately, an occasional high reading is a doubtful indication because, as has been seen, an entirely normal individual may appear in the doctor's surgery with high pressure as a result of rushing to keep the appointment, an altercation in the waiting-room, or simple nervousness. Generally, therefore, it is not until an elevated pressure becomes persistent that the subject is reliably identified and treatment can be contemplated.

INSURANCE

With the capability, made possible by the sphygmomanometer, of measuring blood pressure, doctors were quickly able to link high blood pressure with various health risks. But, although the clinical features of associated illness were soon defined, the inability for a long time to lower blood pressure by treatment placed the emphasis on severe cases—an expression of the view that blood pressure was related to risk only at its more extreme levels.

It was the insurance companies that changed this attitude. From 1910 they began gathering statistics on a vast scale, especially in the United States, concerning the effects of health factors on length of life.

In 1959 and 1961, studies were published covering more than 5 million insured lives, a massive wealth of figures from which it was possible to estimate the normal life expectancy of individuals who had no adverse health factors and to calculate how far this was diminished by factors such as high blood pressure.

The striking fact emerged that, apart from a tiny group of rare cases, levels of blood pressure related continuously to a decreasing scale of life expectancy from low to high pressure—that is to say, those with the lowest pressures could expect the longest lives; those with the highest pressures, the shortest lives; those in between on a graded scale. Any notion of a point dividing harmful from harmless blood pressure levels was now proved wrong. To insist on separate categories, observed one doctor, was to dodge the very issue of timely treatment by which the worst harm could be turned aside.

3

Some Complexities

Those hypertensives who lead normal, vigorous lives thanks to the up-to-date treatment of high blood pressure can be grateful they did not live earlier. During recent years, radical improvements have taken place in the availability of drugs capable of everything short of an actual cure. Countless hypertensive subjects are today living with perfectly normal blood pressure, no different from that of other healthy people of their age, except that they must keep taking the medicine. It is a small chore.

Their grandparents had less luck. In 1914, when insurance companies were wanting blood pressure readings from new clients, a leading authority on hypertension described it as one of the processes in which nature could "not often be thwarted."

Interest in the problem, stimulated by the advent of a practical sphygmomanometer, languished somewhat owing to the lack of an effective controlling agent. In those early days, recommended treatments for lowering blood pressure—some helpful, some less so—included sleep and rest, a vegetarian diet, water therapy, oxygen baths, purging, blood-letting and the application of high-frequency electrical currents. Sufferers were advised on the one hand to take exercise; on the other hand, to conserve their energy.

Some treatment, including radioactive injections and exposure to radium emanation, was dangerous; some was expensive. Because a warm, relaxing climate was thought desirable, patients were urged to winter in Bermuda, Jamaica, Egypt, California, or Florida. Between the world wars, different preparations to lower blood pressure were tried with scant success.

Diagnosis, by contrast, was improved by important work, notably in the field of retinal appearance. By inspecting the retina—the layer of light-sensitive skin behind the eyeball—researchers found that the delicate blood vessels there changed in character at different stages of hypertension. By the simple process of looking into a patient's eyes, the doctor could obtain useful evidence to supplement that of the manometer. Thus, while practical treatment was yet awaited, knowledge of the varying levels of hypertension and the associated problems advanced.

High blood pressure is a major health hazard because people with it are more prone to strokes, heart disease, or kidney failure than people with lower pressure. The importance of modern treatment is that when the pressure is lowered—and in the vast majority of cases it *does* fall—the risks described fall along with it.

What delayed effective treatment until the post-World War II era was the fact that the cause of most hypertension was, and still is, debatable. Instead of knowing what preparations to go for, it was a question of trial and error, of testing various drugs and drug combinations until they worked, then refining and extending them.

As a basis for diagnosis, doctors usually define chronic high blood pressure as one showing a systolic pressure persistently greater than 150 mm and a diastolic pressure persistently greater than 95 mm. Ninety per cent of patients with chronic high blood pressure have what is called "essential" or "enigmatic" hypertension—in other words, the cause of the condition is uncertain.

In the minority of cases where the cause can be ascertained, and may include kidney damage, disease of the endocrine glands, abnormality of the aorta, and other problems, the cure is a specific one. Otherwise, it has been pointed out, hypertension is a purely arbitrary distinction applied to some blood pressures in the higher ranges, the factors involved in its genesis being those involved in determining blood pressure in the overall population.

One conclusion of world research into the mechanisms that regulate blood pressure is that hypertension is not, in its common form, a single so much as a complex problem in which the same result—the high pressure—may be caused by one or more of several defects. This idea accords with established facts. Whereas blood pressure depends clearly on two factors—the resistance of the vessels to the flow of blood through them, and the volume of fluid in the system—the regulation of these involves a complicated interaction among different systems: circulatory, nervous, endocrine, and excretory.

This being so, and each system being influenced not only by each of the others but also by such conditions as the water and salt balance of the body, it can be seen that unraveling the mechanisms controlling blood pressure is no slight task.

INVESTIGATION

For a long time hypertension has been linked in a which-came-first debate involving hardening of the arteries (arteriosclerosis). Both are conditions associated with middle and later years, and they often occur together. In hardening of the arteries, a deposit of fatty material in the wall of the artery leads at length to a loss of that elasticity in the vessel that facilitated the blood flow.

It has been argued that high blood pressure in such a case stems from the resulting effort of the heart to maintain an adequate circulation under the difficulties. It has also been argued, and is now held more probable, that the high blood pressure is the cause of the hardening arteries, although the conditions are not inseparable.

Current medical opinion favors the belief that raised blood pressure stems from a spasm of the lesser arteries, that is, the arterioles. Evidence exists that spasm of the arteries to the kidneys has the effect of producing a substance called *renin* which raises the blood pressure. But the cause of the spasm is not agreed on. One theory is that it is produced by that substance beloved by sports writers, adrenalin. Adrenalin, a hormone excreted by the adrenal glands under conditions of mental and physical pressure, stimulates circulation and muscular action. It can, indeed, produce spasm of the arteries. However, it has never been demonstrated that people with hypertension have an excess of adrenalin in their blood. Nor does the theory explain why some people who live or work under pressure are hypertensive and some are not.

Much recent investigation, including research by teams at the Columbia-Presbyterian and Cornell University Medical Centers, has concentrated on *renin.* An enzyme produced by the kidney, renin is instrumental in the formation of substances found in blood and known as *angiotensins.*

Angiotensins act to raise blood pressure in several ways. For example, they stimulate secretion by the cortex of the adrenal gland of a hormone called *aldersterone,* which promotes water retention through the kidney. The resulting increase of fluid in the circulatory system raises blood pressure.

Angiotensins also stimulate the release by the sympathetic nervous system of a nerve transmitter called *norepinephrine.* The sympathetic nervous system is that part of the body's self-governing apparatus that helps it respond to stress. One of the effects of norepinephrine release is increased blood pressure caused by constriction of the arterioles. Constriction, or conversely dilation, of these small vessels is a major factor determining the amount of pressure needed to force the blood through the circulatory system.

Renin, encouraging angiotensins, is therefore a key substance. What releases it? One stimulus is a drop in the pressure of the blood flowing through the kidney. At this, sufficient renin is produced to raise the pressure. A feedback mechanism ensures that the raised pressure is not maintained above the right level for too long. But if the feedback mechanism is faulty, hypertension may result.

Admittedly, say researchers, many hypertensives appear to have normal renin concentrations—but, because high blood pressure should suppress renin production, in their case "normal" concentrations may be too much.

Here the problem gets really tricky. Observing an abnormal renin release process does not explain the cause of it. The cause may be in the kidney; it may be in the nervous system. Or elsewhere.

Experiments have indicated that the brain, too, is involved in regulating blood pressure. Two areas—the subnucleus medialis, located in the midbrain, and the postrema, in the base of the brain—are relevant. Destruction of these areas has been shown to eliminate blood pressure response to angiotensin.

A special reason for interest in the relationship between the nervous system and hypertension is the common, if scientifically unestablished, belief that stress causes chronic high blood pressure. Stress, as has been noted, can cause temporary increases of pressure. Can high pressure become permanent if stress is present for long periods? It could, suggest experts, if heightened pressure produces chemical or structural changes in blood vessels. And, perhaps significantly, investigators have reported changes in the artery walls of hypertensive animals which, if sustained, might result in further increases of blood pressure.

Another line of inquiry centers on the deficiency of *kinins,* small peptides in the blood that lower pressure by increasing the secretion of water and causing the dilation of blood vessels. The production of kinins involves an enzyme called *kallikrein.* Research at the National Heart, Lung and Blood Institute in the United States, and elsewhere, has indicated that hypertensives secrete less kallikrein in their urine than do people with lower blood pressure.

It has also been noted by American scientists that on the average Black children secrete lower concentrations of kallikrein than white children, even when the Black children have normal blood pressure. The incidence of high blood pressure is known to be much greater in the Black population than among the whites.

Furthermore, the blood pressure levels in families with low kallikrein concentrations have been found to be significantly higher than in those families with greater kallikrein concentrations. Such observations suggest that a biochemical irregularity, perhaps of genetic origin, may predispose some people to the development of hypertension.

It is known that the hereditary factor in hypertension is conspicuous. In about a third of cases, variations in the distribution of blood pressure at large reflect the tendency of children to resemble parents. Some researchers believe it could be nearer two-thirds. And the link is most evident in persons with raised pressures—except for persons with the severest cases who, paradoxically, show the least concordance with their relatives.

Variations between populations are interesting. In terms of the broadest distribution, Western people are far more prone to hypertension than are Eastern people, whereas among a few isolated peoples blood pressures are not only very low but remain stable, or even fall with age. This is true, for instance, of the fish and vegetable eaters of Polynesia and the carnivorous Masai tribe of Africa. One settled, one nomadic, they offer no conspicuous similarities of life style to explain their low blood pressure. It is even more confusing to observe that ethnic groups that *do* resemble the Polynesians or the Masai do not conform to their low age-stable blood pressures. No consistent racial or environmental factor has been identified.

WHO IS VULNERABLE?

Perhaps the least contentious statement about hypertension is that what is known of it is dwarfed by what is not known. Attitudes of doctors to the problem vary considerably, and few assumptions go unchallenged. All the same, some clues to its incidence stand out.

As has been seen, the problem is far less likely to manifest itself in those under the age of forty than those over forty, and it is most likely to appear between fifty and sixty. During the reproductive years it is more common in men than women, after which the incidence is reversed.

Apart from no longer being youthful, the hypertensive subject, it seems, is more likely to be fat than thin, and, curious though it may appear, less likely to have children than persons with normal levels of blood pressure.

The link with obesity is familiar. Tests on a sample of nearly 68,000 people showed an average rise of 2 mm systolic and 3 mm diastolic for each 22 pounds of extra weight—not a dramatic effect. It is known, however, that obese people can achieve markedly lower pressures by reducing their weight.

The relationship between blood pressure and parental status is as intriguing as it is puzzling.The phenomenon fades in the fifth decade, but up to that age the tendency of husbands and wives to have lower pressure if they have children has been established by independent researchers in more than one country. After age fifty the blood pressure of parents and nonparents apparently becomes equal.

According to a further study, coital frequency was not related to blood pressure. Assumptions about the strain of sexual deprivation leading to high blood pressure, like assumptions about the stresses of modern life, often fail to match existing evidence. Although some studies of blood pressure in urban and rural populations have shown higher levels in the former, other studies have shown the opposite. A comparison between mining and rural populations in Wales revealed no difference. Nor does blood pressure seem *consistently* related to occupational physical activity, sleep habits, salt intake, or the amount of cholesterol in the blood.

There *is* an association between the contraceptive pill, the estrogen-progestogen preparation, and raised blood pressure in some cases. The rise, however, is usually slight, and the level reverts to normal three months after the pill is stopped.

The short answer to "who is likely to be hyptertensive?" is "almost anyone."

4

Signs and Symptoms

Doctors hold divergent views on symptoms and hypertension. At one extreme it is held that high blood pressure is symptomless; at the other, that it is largely a symptomatic condition.

Being without symptoms, says the first school, high blood pressure cannot be diagnosed in the usual way by patients presenting themselves to a doctor for relief of symptoms. This is confirmed, goes the argument, by the high proportion of hypertensives known to be receiving no treatment.

Studies based on population samples in the United States, the United Kingdom, and Australia have shown that as many as two-thirds of the hypertensives in these nations remain undiagnosed. By far the greater number of these are males—reflecting, it seems, the tendecy of women to consult their doctors more readily than do men.

Most hypertensives, insists the asymptomatic school, have no more symptoms than otherwise comparable people with lower pressures. Such "traditional" signs as headaches, palpitation, and dizziness occur as frequently in nonhypertensive individuals as in those with high blood pressure. At least, this is so, it is claimed, until patients are told they have high blood pressure, when they may complain more often of symptoms.

Against the skeptics is set a considerable body of medical opinion holding views at the opposite extreme. More than a third of British general practitioners who responded to one inquiry considered that hypertensives *usually* consulted doctors because of symptoms, especially headache and vertigo.

Between these extremes lies the view that although many patients with hypertension—especially mild hypertension—are symptom-free and their hypertension is detected only by routine examination, those with higher pressures not uncommonly have symptoms, including morning headaches, failing vision, breathlessness, buzzing in the ears, and so on.

Few symptoms, agrees one authority, are specific to hypertensive patients, and "it is often difficult to explain their physical basis or relationship to hypertension," but symptoms they are, nonetheless, and they often signal particular phases of hypertension.

Symptoms, signs, associated conditions—however they are regarded—can best be described by those who have experienced them. Here, for example, is one patient's description of the headaches he experienced *before* discovering he was hypertensive and that vanished after the commencement of treatment for that condition:

> The headache was dull but persistent, rooted, it seemed, in the neck with the main discomfort at the back of the head and behind the eyes. For a long time I didn't worry; after all, headaches are commonplace as the result of everyday stress.
>
> But it nagged monotonously and, most depressing, I woke up with it. I'd try to shake it off by taking another nap, but it would still be there when I woke up again.
>
> The only hope of getting rid of it, having got up, was to do as little as possible. Any kind of effort, particularly involving concentration, made things worse. It was a sickening way to start a new day.

In some cases where hypertensives complain of headache the pain diminishes when the victim rises and has breakfast, to return at a later hour. In other cases, it persists through the day and lets up at evening. Or it may continue round the clock—for several days on end, sometimes.

A "bruised feeling" behind the eyes is mentioned by some patients.

> At first the headache gave me perhaps one bad day a week; in the end, a bad one for every good one, though they came in clusters, three or four bad ones in succession, and I spent the others simply washed-out.
>
> It was like living with a hangover, as if you went to bed intoxicated, not a searing pain but blunt and deadening. Any form of noise, hustle, or altercation aggravated it. You just wanted to switch off and be alone.

Others speak of the less-than-alive feeling conveyed by the "hangover" analogy, the nausea that may accompany it, a general sensation of being vulnerable to the world at large.

Many hypertensives first consult a doctor with such signs and claim that the problems largely disappear with lowered blood pressure. A business woman recalled:

> I would be sitting at my desk concentrating on some problem or another, when suddenly I realized my mind had blanked out. There I was practically rigid with concentration and thinking of nothing. I felt sick. My head was aching, and when I put my hands to it the temple was throbbing rapidly.
>
> I had to lie down. There was a settee in the corner. On one occasion I felt so bad I could not walk to it, having instead to go all round the room leaning on the walls.
>
> After that I took a holiday. It was work strain, neurosis, I told myself. The holiday made no difference.
>
> So constant were the headaches that I ended up shuffling about in a kind of daze, a walking cabbage until, at last, my sister tackled me. "You're forty-six," she said one day, "and you act like an old woman. You're barely alive. What on earth's the matter? Who is your doctor?" I told her. She drove me round and he informed me my blood pressure was sky-high.
>
> It was the last thing I'd have thought of. I didn't even know what hypertension was.

This type of patient, intelligent enough to think the problem neurotic in origin, may put off visiting a doctor for far too long. Yet it is simple and quick to check the blood pressure. Such patients, runs the argument for routine screening, should be diagnosed and treated earlier.

PALPITATIONS

There is no more reason for supposing that an obtrusive heartbeat means hypertension than for thinking that a headache does—or for worrying if one's heart thumps. Since normally this most vital and constant friend toils unheeded, it seems churlish to object to being reminded of it now and then. Yet, as every doctor knows, people do object and some get most alarmed. Commonly, this occurs as palpitations, the result of overstimulated nerves or anxiety, often experienced and first noticed in bed at night. The greater the worry at the discovery, the more persistent becomes the throb. The answer is to stop worrying. Sit up and the thumping, throbbing beat that can be so frightening will probably stop. It will calm down in its own time. In any case, a healthy heart can pound for weeks without being harmed.

Hypertensives sometimes first consult their doctors with palpitations, among other signs. Recalled one patient:

> Before treatment my heart used to thump like a boys' band. Sometimes I couldn't sleep for it. Whatever position I tried to rest in it seemed that my heart, or one pulse or another, kept up the hammering. Since treatment, it is far rarer, and never as obtrusive as it used to be.

The same man also experienced physical tension in his arms and limbs when he tried to rest.

> For a while, I'd not be conscious it was happening. Then, perhaps lying in bed before sleeping, I'd notice my ankles clamped to-

> gether. Unlocking them, I'd tell myself to relax, to stop tightening up.
>
> But it was as if they were magnetized, irresistibly attracted. Back they would go together and, in the end, it was more effort to keep them apart than to let them have their own way, so I would give up.

Treatment for hypertension reduced both the palpitations and muscular tension. The patient was helped to relax properly.

GIDDINESS

Giddiness is sometimes linked with hypertension and can signify changes of blood pressure. Another patient told his doctor of twice feeling momentarily giddy before commencing treatment for high blood pressure, both incidents occurring on what he called his better days. Once, sitting beside his wife in the car waiting for a red traffic light to change, he felt strangely lightheaded and realized the light was green without his having observed the change. The sensation went as abruptly as it came. He felt fine again. In fact, although it may be associated with elevated blood pressure, giddiness more often occurs when high pressure transiently falls, maybe caused by hot weather, taking sleeping pills, or some other reason. It was hot in the car. Perhaps in this instance the patient's soaring pressure, undiscovered at that time, had taken a brief descent. Certainly that was true, according to her doctor, of a woman hypertensive who had spent a sun-worshipping interlude at a beach resort and found the world spinning when she sat up. "Luckily my husband was with me. I stretched out again, this time in the shade, and it went away," she said.

Indeed, for the hypertensive a giddy spell is more often a sign of reassuring development than otherwise. And, of course, for most people giddiness has nothing to do with high blood pressure. In most cases it is caused by no more than bending while gardening or washing hair, jumping up too quickly in the morning, by wax on the eardrum, as a passing concomitant of the menopause, and so on.

Another phenomenon sometimes associated with hypertension, and which can indicate changing pressure, is whistling or ringing in the ears, known as *tinnitus*. Like giddiness, this may indicate movement of the blood pressure either way. It can be a welcome signal to those who experience it after treatment.

EYESIGHT

Untreated hypertensives may sometimes experience impaired vision. One patient said:

> My sight became blurred and I found difficulty reading small print. Considering the headaches I suffered, especially if I taxed my eyes, I concluded I needed glasses.
>
> After the normal tests of vision, these were prescribed for reading and close work, and were an aid. At about this time I enjoyed a lessening in the incidence of headaches and thought the glasses had done the trick.

When, after a prolonged respite, the headaches became bad again, this man returned to the optician for more help. An optician is not trained to investigate health problems. Tests indicated that the lenses should be changed, and this was done. Twice over a span of years the lenses were adjusted, the second time not just for close use but for middle distance, TV, and driving. Even so, concentrated visual activity was a strain. The headaches became prolonged. It was an effort to focus, and driving was an ordeal. Diagnosis and treatment of the hypertension followed.

> The most extraordinary of all things as my blood pressure normalized was the restoration of good sight. I'd not realized how bad my eyes had become until objects were bright and distinct again.

> I can't describe the pleasure of rediscovering vivid colors after the greyness that had dulled everything. I once bought an old, begrimed oil painting in a sale and watched a picture restorer wipe over it with a cleansing agent. As he wiped, the filth of years dissolved and brilliant hues emerged from a murky monotone.
>
> That was exactly what it was like to see afresh after the treatment. For years I had depended on glasses. I haven't worn them since my blood pressure was controlled.

UNHEEDED SIGNALS

Many independent, hard-working people will tolerate such indications of stress and tension for long periods rather than consider failing in their responsibilities as breadwinners and family guardians. After all, they may argue, everybody gets headaches. To stop work for headaches is impractical. Moreover, warning signals, in cases where they do arise, may develop insidiously—a bad day now and then at the beginning—so that the victim becomes inured, learns to cope as well as possible.

Maybe he has the kind of job where he can ride out the worst moments at a slack pace, making up work when he feels better, perhaps in his own time. Maybe he can get out of his place of work on some kind of errand when he feels below par, be in the fresh air. Maybe he will resort increasingly to aspirin, or some other analgesic, to screen the problem. Recalled a woman who worked with an accounting firm:

> I would get to my desk and read the letters. If I felt worse, I would leave an excuse in the office and slip out to a nearby snack bar for a cup of coffee and an aspirin. With luck, sitting quietly for ten minutes would help a little.
>
> Then I would return to the office and take things very gently for an hour or two, catching up over lunchtime, or taking work home at night. I got it done, but it became harder and harder to keep up to a normal appearance—and the amount of aspirin I swallowed was phenomenal.

Maybe, at last, mere tactics do not suffice—it comes to strategy.

One man, a skilled mechanic in line for promotion at a large factory, left to set up on his own doing car repairs. He said:

> I simply had to find a way of getting round the hours when I didn't feel up to it. By working for myself, I thought I would solve the problem: make the time up evenings and weekends. I suppose I just didn't have the temperament to be my own boss. Or the capital. Without a steady paycheck I fretted and felt worse.

On the other hand, a commercial artist who left his firm to freelance was so successful the orders piled up. The more frantically he strove to cope with them, the worse he felt. He recalled: "The point is, at the time you blame the things you know about: the worry, the pressure, the overwork. You know you feel worse the more they mount up. What you don't know is that beneath it your blood pressure is creeping up."

In an extreme case the point can be reached where the subject, when not working mechanically, has almost no life. The wife of one such patient recalled her anxiety:

> You could say that my husband *existed*, and that was all. We had enjoyed going to the movies, but now he would want to leave after five or ten minutes, saying the film was rubbish. In fact, watching the screen made him feel bad. If we stayed, I would notice him sitting with his eyes closed.
>
> In the past we had liked to drive out to a little inn we knew for a quiet drink. Now, the least drop of alcohol made his head ache, and he had grown too introverted to talk to strangers. Even the idea of having friends in, or going out to them, upset him.
>
> I thought it must be mind over matter: that he felt unwell because he just did not wish to do these things. I didn't realize that he *dared* not—that he would have loved to go to a movie, for a drink, in the assurance that he would feel all right.
>
> At one point I decided it was my fault; that I did not suit him. After twenty years of successful marriage! It could have broken our relationship had he not seen a doctor at long last.

5

Treatment

Symptoms, when they exist with common or enigmatic hypertension, can usually be relieved rapidly. Although this is important for sufferers, it is not the main aim of treatment in such cases, and clearly not so in the larger number of cases, which are symptomless. The primary and continuing aim of treatment is to eliminate the risks associated with high blood pressure so far as possible for the rest of the subject's life.

"A vast weight of evidence," Dr. Julian Tudor Hart has written in his prize-winning paper on the management of high blood pressure in general practice, "supports the view that the harmful effects of hypertension derive almost wholly from sustained raised pressure in the arterial lumen, and are reversed by its sustained reduction."

The means now available, for the most part pills, involve the patient in only minor inconvenience, and it should be understood that, once started, treatment is likely to be for life.

Two principles are important:

1. Persons under treatment will not achieve the best results unless they persevere conscientiously with the regimen. Ineffective treatment caused by casual compliance is unfortunately widespread among patients.

2. Persons left untreated as borderline cases should report to the doctor as directed for pressure readings in case treatment should become, with time, advisable.

Since the cause of most hypertension is uncertain, there is not so much a precise treatment as a range of options doctors can employ in the light of what they know of an individual case. Cases vary in severity and complication. Age, temperament, and general health weigh in the balance, but most hypertensives live perfectly normally under treatment, with perhaps a modicum of self-restraint. Such restraints include the reduction of weight where excessive, limitations on smoking and drinking alcohol, and ample rest.

Very fat people with mild hypertension may bring their blood pressure within acceptable levels simply by reducing weight—if "simple" is the right word. Unsustained weight reduction will not do.

Another straightforward, if unpalatable, regime with pressure-lowering properties is a low-salt diet. It is necessary for the salt restriction to be so severe to obtain a small reduction in pressure that the treatment is usually combined with other pressure-reducing treatments.

In the 1940s, before drug treatment for hypertension became dependable, there was a vogue for a rice, sugar, and fruit diet almost free of sodium. Some results were good, but few people were prepared to live on such an unvaried diet for very long.

DRUG PREPARATIONS

Not all the drugs used against hypertension are new discoveries. One, *rauwolfia,* also known as a tranquillizer, comes from a large climbing plant recognized for centuries in the East for its healing properties. Rauwolfia grows widely in India, Malaya, Ceylon, and Burma. It is now chiefly utilized in the form of *reserpine,* an alkaloid obtained from the plant root. So popular has been its use to treat fevers, nervous problems, and insomnia in the regions of its origin that one manufacturer sold 50 million tablets of it in India in ten years. Reserpine is thought to reduce blood pressure by depleting transmitter stores in the nervous system.

Also of plant extraction, though from the West, are the *veratrum* derivatives from what is commonly called poke or green hellebore, a perennial herb found in Europe and America. It has bright yellowish-green flowers, two to four on a stem, and large leaf-like bracts. Both green hellebore and its relative, black hellebore, the "Christmas rose," contain properties poisonous to animals feeding on them. As with rauwolfia, the extract used in the treatment of high blood pressure, *veratrine,* is taken from the root. Performing both as a sedative and a depressant of the heart and nervous system, it is a powerful pressure-lowering agent, but it is used rarely now owing to the nausea and vomiting caused in many cases.

Another interesting drug, *hydrallazine,* has been limited in its application by the unpleasant side-effects—including headaches, flushing and palpitations—often encountered when used in higher doses. Its direct dilating action on the blood vessels makes it particularly appropriate to use when swift action is required to reduce excessive fluid.

GANGLION BLOCKADE

The era of effective drug treatment of hypertension began in 1950, and that of widely acceptable treatment began in 1960. Between these dates, a decade of striking advances in the discovery of pressure-lowering agents was hampered by problems of application and side-effects.

A significant step forward was the introduction of ganglion-blocking drugs—that is, drugs that act by producing a block in the ganglia (the knots on the nerves from which the nerve fibres radiate) of the autonomic nervous system, lessening stimulant action. Such substances had first been noted when it was found that the substance tetraethyl ammonium chloride blocked the stimulant action of nicotine.

In 1949 researchers in this field carried out the first clinical trials, including that of pentane iodide (known as C.5) by administering the drugs to themselves. In the recumbent position they found little effect on blood pressure from C.5, but one doctor promptly fainted from the drop in his pressure when he stood up. When treatment became widespread, countless hypertensives were to experience a similar response to postural variation—caused by the inhibition of the body's normal mechanism for adjusting to such changes.

Meanwhile, initial skepticism toward C.5 and C.6 (hexamethonium) was banished in 1950 by the report of a New Zealand doctor that the use of these drugs on hypertensive patients had already produced remarkable successes. Ganglion-blocking medicine, the advance guard of a major assault on hypertension, had made its mark.

In the 1950s ganglion blockers did good work, but they were tricky to use efficiently and side-effects—including loss of saliva, constipation, and postural complications—did not endear them to all patients.

ADRENERGETIC BLOCKING DRUGS

The ganglion blockers were unselective in their action, and in the late 1950s the first of the more selective neurone-blocking drugs were tested. Focusing the blockade where it was effective, they eliminated a lot of the unpleasantness of ealier side-effects and signaled an era of mass treatment which, by 1973, was topping 9,250,000 prescriptions a year for antihypertensive drugs in Britain alone.

To the drugs of the 1960s—*debrisoquine, bethanidine, guanethidine*—was added in the 1970s the so-called beta blockers—*propranolol, oxprenolol, pindolol, alprenolol, practolol*—extending a by-now diverse armory.

DIURETICS

Among the well-established weapons against hypertension were the diuretics. Diuretics, substances that promote the excretion of urine, had always presented a way of reducing body salt without dieting. Until 1957, however, potent quantities had to be given by injection. The breakthrough to oral treatment came with a preparation called *chlorothiazide.* Thiazide diuretics have a mild pressure-lowering action aside from their diuretic property, and they can safely be combined with another drug as a "background" treatment. As well as a stable dose response, they offer the advantage of reducing blood pressure irrespective of posture, so that sudden drops in level are not experienced by the patient after exercise or standing up. This makes them especially useful to the elderly or infirm on mild treatment.

Today, the full list of antihypertensive drugs is too long to give here, but clonidine and methyldopa stand apart in their interest and are worth note.

CLONIDINE AND METHYLDOPA

Both clonidine and methyldopa operate by unusual modes that are not fully understood. Clonidine, sometimes used when migraine headache is involved, is thought to achieve its pressure-lowering effect by direct action on the vasomotor center in the brain stem. The vasomotor center controls the constriction and dilation of blood vessels.

Methyldopa's action, possibly disturbing the nerve transmitter noradrenaline, is as obscure, but the drug has a popular record despite its tendency to bring on tiredness unless used in small quantities.

Most drugs present problems of some kind for some people, so the option of alternatives briefly indicated here is comforting. Selection of the best drug, or drugs, for the individual may depend on other conditions to which he is susceptible —for instance, some preparations are not suitable for those prone to asthma—or for which he already receives drugs. People requiring permanent drug treatment for several serious disorders clearly present doctors with difficulties. These are not insuperable, although treatment for marginal hypertension might not be recommended in such cases.

Doctors are not usually as anxious to place the elderly on pressure-lowering drugs as they are others with high pressures. People who are fit at sixty-five and over and who have high blood pressure—and there are many of them—are probably naturally tough to begin with.

Before drugs are prescribed, a routine medical examination will have eliminated the possibility of the less common causes of high blood pressure. Sometimes persons recommended to treatment are worried by the notion of hypertension, particularly if new to it.

As one patient, successfully treated, explained

> Most health problems a lot of people get are talked about: arthritis, diabetes, the familiar things. They crop up in conversation. There are books in the library about having coronaries, recovering from strokes, and so on. But hypertension—I'd heard nothing, read nothing. I wish I had. I would have been reassured had I known that there were more than 11 million visits to doctors that year for high blood pressure.

Familiarity reduces needless apprehension.

Remember that in the great majority of cases hypertension is simply a variant of normal blood pressure; treatment is a wise precautionary measure, and no more.

SURGERY

As well as drugs, there are two other kinds of treatment. One of them, surgery, is mainly of historical interest. The most common surgical operation performed for the relief of hypertension before the advent of modern drugs was sympathectomy, a procedure involving cutting the sympathetic nerve fibers to the abdominal organs, which were thought to be responsible for the impulses leading to spasm of the arteries. This procedure was sometimes extended by complete or partial adrenalectomy.

A review of operations on the eve of the drug era must have discouraged sympathectomy, regardless of the effectiveness of ganglion-blocking drugs. In the United States, only 8 per cent of patients subjected to the operation had normal levels of blood pressure five years afterward, and only a further 13 per cent showed any decrease of former levels. And many of these cases had been relatively mild ones.

In England, where operations were confined to severe cases, no more than eleven in eighty patients were found to have gained any lasting fall in pressure.

The other and more relevant treatment centers on controlling the stresses and tensions in the patient's life. Here, the doctor's influence is limited—we must consider the problem in a broader light.

6

Social Stress

Many assumptions are made about stress in hypertension, but few have been proven. There is no shortage of causes for complaint in modern life: the pace and noise, bad housing, high mortgage rates, unemployment all bring strain and unhappiness. But how relevant are they to hypertension?

Hypertension's incidence is lower in Eastern communities where people live in mud dwellings and where famine, flood, and destitution are endemic. Are these less stressful than noise and mortgage rates?

In Western societies, excessive overtime, shiftwork, and the line speeds demanded in modern factories are suspected causes of hypertension. Yet the incidence of high blood pressure is lower in some places where peasants still slave incessantly to subsist. Is that less stressful than working shifts for a good wage?

The problem, think some researchers, may be related to social change. Groups with raised blood pressure, they say, show increased tension and conflict owing to individual failure to adapt to the environment. Communities with unchanging conditions, however hard these may be, are more likely to show low pressures. Where the habitual life-style of a population is upset by change, runs the hypothesis, a proportion of its membership affected by the challenge to adjust will develop hypertension.

Strong and repeatedly threatening stimuli, observe psychiatrists, may result from changing social conditions such as those in rapidly growing or modernizing cities. An example occurs when the neighborliness of long-standing slum areas is replaced by impersonal development. It could be the same where small country communities are faced with "progress."

Especially challenged by the problems of adaption are the middle-aged. By middle-age, it is claimed, people have come to depend on established social values which, in a changing world, may be beset on all sides. Under such circumstances, suggests one theory, people sustain repetitive pressure-raising shocks to the nervous system (i.e., hypothalmic arousals). Such signals may lead eventually to permanent high blood pressure. This theory at least accords with the fact that hypertensives often experience transient episodes of high blood pressure before the persistent stage.

In one case the subject, a talented musician, had from youth coveted a career with a major orchestra, but, marrying young, had been obliged to abandon the pursuit of art and take a secure job to keep his family. Working as a salesman, he made music in his spare time with an amateur quartet. Eventually the job became increasingly irksome to him, he developed headaches and, as routine insurance medical examinations disclosed, transient high blood pressure. The latter meant nothing to him, and time passed. Then his luck changed. Following a chance introduction, he was offered a full-time professional position with a viable if less than illustrious musical ensemble. He was overjoyed at last to have a foot on the ladder of his ambition. The headaches disappeared. For a couple of years, while improving and gaining experience, he remained content. Then the compulsion to climb stirred. The ensemble no longer stretched his talents. Rehearsals became an ordeal, and he longed to get away from it. The headaches returned; blood pressure rose again. Finally, casting about for opportunities, he was invited to join a provincial orchestra of distinction where, for a while, he was again content and free of symptoms. But, in turn, he outgrew the new post; the symptoms came back. Thus, in a now-familiar sequence—frustration and discomfort released by a step forward; fulfilment until frustration built up again—his life continued.

Today, as a senior member of a world-renowned orchestra, he has reached his goal; treatment has controlled the hypertension that became severe in middle-age. He is satisfied. The case is interesting, not only as an example of hypertensive episodes leading to the chronic state, but because the symptoms clearly coincide with those periods when the subject was most at dissonance with his surroundings but *least* taxed at work.

There is much doubt about the ways in which emotional processes increase blood pressure, but some investigation has suggested that the action may come about quite differently from the widely assumed notion that it is an alerting or tuning-in response to immediate environmental stimuli. In fact, according to Malcolm J. MacCullock of the Department of Psychiatry at Liverpool University, elevated pressure may result from the organism's attempt to *limit* response to surroundings, rather than to heighten vigilance. According to this theory, increases in blood pressure and heart rate produce a "stimulus barrier" that restricts sensory input to the brain, while decreases of pressure and heart rate produce "a less impermeable barrier." Supporting experiments showed that both heart rate and blood pressure rose during tasks that required the subject to think rather than be predominantly vigilant. Most subjects lowered their blood pressure during "environmental intake."

But when the subject wished *to reduce his sensory input, he raised his blood pressure and heart rate. Conditions of vigilance in which he* desired *to pay attention to the external world reduced his blood pressure and heart rate.* Such findings are quite contrary to widely accepted theory.

If, then, it is believed that episodic rises in blood pressure lead by repetition to sustained hypertension, and if it is believed that such rises may in part be nature's way of blocking out unwanted aspects of environment, it follows that the disruption of societies by noise pollution, new housing schemes, new highways, and so on is a major medical responsibility.

The matter, of course, is a much wider one.

When an organism undertakes any new task, or is subjected to any stimulus to which it is not accustomed, changes occur in such vital functions as sweating, blood pressure, and heart rate. And life today is remorseless in its novelty—new ways of living, working, traveling. One wonders if the novelty is always worth the cost of more stress.

WORK AND STRESS

Hard work, our grandfathers used to say, never killed anyone. Axioms change like other fashions. A middle-aged hypertensive, reporting for a checkup, was told by the receptionist at the clinic: "Hypertension? Someone's been working too hard, then!"

The patient laughed. "Hard work never killed anyone."

"They all say that," the girl said cheerfully.

Is work a culprit? For those who have retired, or are on the point of retirement, the problem of relating hypertension and its treatment to the demands of a job is academic. The domestic tasks of retirement accommodate a benign routine. But for others the question is a crucial one. In many cases, economic survival depends on work, and, as one doctor puts it, "to tell a hypertensive patient, in effect, to put his feet up and worry how his dependents are going to manage may be as bad as insisting he work all hours."

In our grandfathers' day, work for most was manually demanding. There is no evidence to link manual work, within normal bounds, with high blood pressure. On the other hand, it guarantees no immunity from the stresses that can occur in all work—those associated with difficulties, time pressures, personality conflicts, among others.

Stress is widely assumed to go with certain types of job, but if it is true that a lot of people who get hypertension work in demanding fields, so do a lot of people who do not get hypertension. Indeed, many function at their best under pressure and difficulty, or even crisis, some deliberately seek such challenges.

A retired journalist, asked why he had given up writing when at last he had the leisure to tackle a favorite subject, answered: "I can't do it without a deadline hanging over me. The inspiration's gone now the pressure's off."

Can a source of stimulation and satisfaction also be a source of stress? Many resourceful, competent hypertensives seem at face value to be the least vulnerable of people to work-related stress. As the wife of one patient expressed her puzzlement:

> He had always appeared at his best working flat-out, bright-eyed, vigorous. If anything, it seems to be the time off that gets him down. He likes to finish one job and have the next lined up to start right away—not just any job, the most difficult he can get. There is a joke at the firm that if a job is impossible it will keep my husband happy until he has completed it. He never found pleasure in an easy task, nor in taking his time over a hard one.
>
> He works the way some people climb mountains or sail oceans: because he has the talent and relishes the achievement. I can't remember that he ever looked harassed. His colleagues do. Some look permanently fraught—but *they* didn't get hypertension and he did.

Perhaps work was not a factor. Or if it was, it was more subtle than met the eye.

Hypertension is not consistently related to stress symptoms, but "it is probably in psychosocial sensory input," writes

Julian Tudor Hart in his study of high blood pressure, "that most of the so far unspecified causation will be found." Since most people spend a major part of their lives working, it seems a fruitful area for investigation.

Unfortunately it is difficult to measure blood pressure while the subject is working. Techniques for continuous, or semicontinuous recording under everyday conditions may eventually provide useful data. Even so, the complexity of human behavior will make evaluation difficult.

Meanwhile, perhaps most people will continue to complain about the necessity of working while deriving more satisfaction from work than they might admit, until retirement brings the point home.

If it is true that trying to blot out the disagreeable is more likely to raise blood pressure than striving for the desirable, maybe work as such is indeed innocent, and the objective of work satisfaction even more important than widely realized.

And if work per se is not culpable, perhaps the wrong person in a job might be. In which case the hypertensive who finds his, or her, work disagreeable should perhaps think harder about switching occupations.

In the case of the dedicated person, a little less ardor may be advisable—not because the work itself is stressful, but because the inevitable frustrations experienced by the devoted worker may be a source of stress.

7

Starting to Reduce Blood Pressure

Before undergoing treatment for hypertension the patient must understand that, once started, the treatment will be continuous and probably permanent. Unless the undertaking is conscientious, it is pointless. In fact, a casual, spasmodic approach to taking pressure-lowering drugs may be worse than nothing, for unstable levels of blood pressure are the least desired.

Apart from taking the pills prescribed, the hypertensive patient will be committed to regular medical checks. At first, owing to the variability of response to the drugs, these check-ups will be fairly frequent, then at longer intervals depending on the stability and level of blood pressure achieved. Two points the doctor will be keeping an eye on are the long-term tolerance the body may develop to some drugs, which may require an increased dosage, and such side-effects as may require attention.

Swallowing a few tablets each day and going for a blood pressure reading perhaps once in three months is a slight inconvenience to set against the advantages of living with a healthier level of blood pressure. Many people, especially on low doses of the drugs, will notice no effect on their personal lives.

When side-effects *are* encountered, the commonest are relatively trivial and of diminishing inconvenience as the patient grows accustomed to a new regime. Tiredness is one complaint, a weakness that may come on quickly, and as quickly go. According to one patient, a farmer's wife:

> I found myself in the beginning stopping in the day to put my feet up for half an hour or so. I had never done such a thing—always led a hectic life getting the men off, feeding them, and so on. A farm's a busy place. Now, I just felt weak from time to time.

Gradually, her disability passed. The hypertension had been severe, and to be free of the constant headaches she had experienced was such a relief that the tiredness did not worry her. "I was wide-awake mentally, fully conscious of the world again at long lost. It was haytime. I remember. It all looked and smelled wonderful."

The drugs used in the relief of hypertension begin to work rapidly—almost miraculously, it seems, to those who have suffered badly from symptoms associated with high blood pressure. In such cases, the early phase of treatment can be dramatic—a transition between two lives.

Thus, a self-employed technician in his middle years said:

> It was rather like replacing a beat-up old car with something new but of less power. Things were marvelous—not waking up with those dreaded headaches; the restored clarity of vision; atmosphere like wine again instead of like gray smog. On the other hand, I was a bit worried about feeling tired. I seemed to need a lot of rest.
>
> When I thought of the work piling up, apprehension nagged. It seemed I might have lost the old thrust and drive. My doctor said a few weeks of rest would do me no harm. I suppose I had become a bit of a work addict. Now I simply sat out in a deckchair, lounged around, adapted to running on less steam.
>
> I'd go to bed early, read until I dozed off. I slept a lot—wonderful sleep, knowing I would wake up like a normal person, with a clear head. At regular intervals I took the drug. Soon afterwards, my ears would whistle—quite softly, like an off-tune radio or a kettle beginning to boil. It became a familiar and welcome sound. The pressure was falling, I thought. That was a good sound!

Returning to work with new confidence, he paced himself through the day, stopping at a determined hour—something he had not done for many years.

> Previously, I would have worked on late until the job in hand was finished, or at least until the trickiest part of a job was done. Now I knocked off early and forgot work until the next day.
>
> Eventually, as the treatment progressed, the tiredness wore off and I worked later, though always to a fixed hour, calling the time myself instead of letting the job dictate—avoiding the urge to solve problems and complete tasks before letting up. Few things, I decided, were so important they would not keep until morning, when I was fresh.
>
> As a result, I feel well and relaxed, with time to enjoy life. My blood pressure is low, and there have been no other side-effects. The fact is, I get through as much work as I ever did.

POSTURAL VARIATIONS

Regaining the physical equilibrium that, for some, may be mildly upset by treatment is often a matter of perseverance, of giving the system time to adjust itself. The system is remarkably adaptable. For most patients the upsets are negligible. Others may have to live for a while with unfamiliar quirks of behavior from a body whose habits they thought they had learned to the smallest idiosyncrasy long ago. It can be surprising and intriguing, like finding new facets in an old friend. It can reveal, for example, just how unusually a simple operation such as sitting up or lying down can affect one if the physiological processes one takes for granted are modified.

Blockading drugs tend to produce a lower blood pressure in the standing than in the supine posture, particularly on rising from bed in the morning. It is normal for cardiac output to decrease in the upright position, and for blood pressure to be kept level by compensatory constriction of the blood vessels. Blocking drugs may inhibit vasoconstriction and lead to an abrupt fall in pressure when the patient stands up.

The result may be a swimming head or a black-out. One patient recalls:

> Several times, getting up from bed to go to the bathroom, I fainted. I hadn't been under treatment long and I didn't think—just jumped up in the normal way. Next moment I was coming round on the bathroom floor. You don't always stop to reflect when you are half awake, but I learned the lesson in the end and got up, when I had to, in less haste.

In effect, fainting assures a resumption of the horizontal position and consciousness. But, rather than risk a bruise, sit down if the head swims and save a fall. Better still, take a simple tip: Get up from bed in easy stages. Sit up against the pillows for a minute—longer, if it seems necessary. Slip the legs out and sit on the edge of the bed a moment. *Then* get up.

It will cost only a minute or two; it may save a knock; and it is worth pausing, anyway, to be thankful for falling pressure after living with the reverse for any length of time.

Be careful for a while *after* rising in the morning. Standing, after sitting down to breakfast or an early-morning coffee, may cause light-headedness or dizziness. Another woman patient found that getting out of her car made her head swim:

> There was no newspaper delivery on a Sunday and, when breakfast was over, I used to drive to collect the papers. Each time, it was the same: I would get out of the car and into the shop without trouble. Then, as I stood waiting, I'd feel faint and have to rest against the counter or the door-jamb. It quickly passed and happened to me only on those mornings when I went out early for the papers. The car seat was low. I suppose getting out of it was much like getting out of bed a second time.

DRUGS AND EXERCISE

Those who experience tiredness in the early days of treatment can often adapt without great difficulty. Around the house, going shopping, at the office—day-to-day life is taken in the stride again. Activities of a more strenuous nature may be difficult.

Untreated hypertensives are accustomed to a rise in blood pressure when they exert themselves. Those on blockading drugs may find that their pressure drops when they exercise, and they feel weak. For this reason, a doctor may prescribe a different type of drug for a patient who depends on strenuous physical work for his livelihood.

On the other hand, when strenuous exercise plays a less crucial part in a person's life, some inconvenience in, say, gardening or athletic activity may on balance be justified.

The experience of a middle-aged gardening enthusiast is not untypical:

> I felt so good in all other respects with the treatment that I could scarcely credit what happened at first when I wanted to cut the hedge. True, I had left it a while and it had got a bit out of hand, but I had never thought anything of the job—a few hours. Now, I had barely started when my arms weakened and operating the clippers became a strain. Lifting them to cut above my shoulders was an ordeal. It seemed ridiculous. I could not have been working more than five minutes. Taking a short rest on the stepladder, I found that my arms soon regained strength. But a few minutes of clipping and they were pulp again.
>
> Later, I tried to scythe between my apple trees. Three or four minutes and I was all-in. I soon recovered, but just as soon needed a rest again. Before the treatment for hypertension I could have scythed all morning without a break. I told my doctor and he urged me to persevere with the exercise.

Provided there is no medical reason to avoid exertion, perseverance is important. For one thing, exercise helps to eliminate unwanted flab and preserve the arteries, heart, and other organs in good shape. For another, physical exertion helps many people to relax mentally, to shed the stress of daily brain work.

And, a third point, failing the determination to exercise there is no call on some muscles to do other than lose condi-

there is no call on some muscles to do other than lose condition, which is a pity, for the body will adapt in time to the problem of exertion. Recalled the gardener:

> I was painfully long-winded the first season. It took me all summer, in my spare time, to mow ground I should have finished in a fortnight. I felt like quitting, hiring someone. Instead, I pushed myself, taking short rests, working in labored bursts. Next year, the work was easier. And again the third season. I just kept at it, gradually gaining in endurance. Today, I'd tackle any manual job I could do before, and I'm overall fitter than I used to be, despite increased age.

Generally, doctors are less adamant than they used to be about protracted rest, but they do counsel relaxation as far as possible. Until familiar with the treatment it is wise for the patient to avoid rush. If it is necessary to travel to work, get up early enough to allow time for lingering over breakfast and getting dressed. Leave that last-minute dash to others and proceed in a relaxed style.

Most hypertensive subjects are of a mature age, able to use the advantages of maturity—experience, savviness—to do things the calm way.

In most cases where the side-effects of drugs are encountered, it must be emphasized that they are slight—a dry mouth, chilly feet, a tendency to constipation—and pass off with time. In the fewer cases where effects are less tolerable, they are reversible by changing to other medicines in the formidable armory available for use against hypertension.

With some drugs the effects of postural change and weakness are most noticeable within a short time of taking the dose. Then they pass off. If the immediate result of medication is at all debilitating, it may be a simple matter to arrange the doses to coincide with restful, or at least sedentary periods in the routine. This will not inconvenience those whose work is not physical. Mental activity is not impaired.

ALCOHOL

It may not be advisable to drink within a given time of taking the drugs prescribed. Ask the doctor if in any doubt.

INADVERTENT OVERDOSING

It is not difficult, especially when one is tired or busy, to forget that a pill has already been taken and to take a second one. People on pressure-lowering drugs are sometimes frightened on discovering, or imagining, they have done this. They need not be. In the event of feeling dizzy, lie down until the sensation passes. Raising the feet on a pillow or cushion may be helpful.

SLEEPING

When higher blood pressure is evident in a supine posture, it is sometimes helpful to raise the head of the bed some inches on blocks. Alternatively, raise the mattress toward the head by putting cushions under it, and sleep on higher pillows.

Again, ask the doctor if in doubt.

Remember:

There are different types of antihypertensive drugs, and they work in different ways. The same advice is not applicable to all of them.

The essential requirements for effective control are conscientious and continued adherence to a doctor's instructions, and regular checkups.

Treatment will reduce and stabilize blood pressure; it will not banish the problem in the sense that treatment may be stopped when the pressure is satisfactory. Neglect it and hypertension will tend to reassert itself.

Antihypertensive treatment is not short-term. If the objective is defined as attaining the best health possible with the minimum disruption of normal life, then this is a goal to be worked for patiently, through an understanding of the individual case in terms both of medical observation and self-experience. It is a long-term enterprise.

8

Stress and Tension

If it is not certain that psychological stress can actually cause hypertension, there is no doubt that it raises the blood pressure. It follows that to embark on drug treatment while doing nothing to reduce stresses and tensions is to ask more of medication than necessary.

Some stress of a broad environmental nature has been mentioned, much perhaps unavoidable without social change. Other stresses are more personal. The cause often seems trivial, yet, as the sales of sedatives and tranquillizers testify, the spread of stress-related illness is formidable.

To understand how anxiety may affect blood pressure one must consider what experts on behavior call the "fear reflex." At a primitive level, anxiety is essential to survival, for it prepares the body to fight or run in the face of threat. A nonanxious rabbit would not live long, nor would humanity have survived its early history without fear. Anxiety and fear work for survival on a basis that is partly reflex, that is, automatic. The region of the brain responsible for this response (as opposed to the "thinking" part of survival) is the *hypothalamus.*

The *cerebral cortex* takes care of the "thinking" skills. While the cerebral cortex is occupied with conscious thought, a network of nerves governed by the hypothalamus supervises the automatic functions that sustain life.

Every minute, the heart contracts between sixty and ninety times as it pumps blood, the lungs expand and deflate in accord with signals from the chest muscles and diaphragm, food is digested when appropriate. None of these functions is dependent on instructions from the "thinking" brain. The bodily system responsible for such basic functions is known as the *autonomic nervous system.* Its dependence, vital for survival, can raise problems. For example, being for most practical purposes beyond command of the "thinking" brain, the autonomic nervous system cannot consciously be ordered to behave in a given way. Or rather, it can be ordered but probably it will not obey, as anyone knows who has told himself (or herself) to calm down, and could not.

If the autonomic nervous system could be controlled by willpower—as can, say, the movement of arms and legs—people could go some way toward controlling blood pressure by simple thought. But the system, designed for independence, has its own controls: (1) the *sympathetic* branch, concerned with the speeding up or energy-expending side of operations, and (2) the opposing *parasympathetic* branch, concerned with energy conservation or the slowing down of basic functions.

These two branches strive for balance. When a threat looms, the sympathetic branch takes command, and the system puts the body in a state of readiness to do battle or run for safety. The fear reflex has stimulated the fight-or-flight mechanism. Now, heart rate and blood pressure are boosted, likewise the speed of respiration, so that the brain and limbs are kept plentifully supplied with adequately oxygenated blood. Adrenalin is poured into the blood stream so that extra sugar is released for muscle energy. At the same time, blood is drained from irrelevant areas such as the digestive tract and sent to the running and fighting muscles. The clotting speed of the blood is enhanced in case of injury.

All these are vital to survival in a fight-or-flight situation. Having fought or fled, the body has discharged its preparedness, and the parasympathetic branch restores calm as a natural course. The heart slows down, blood pressure falls, the flow of blood no longer favors special muscles.

Such is the mechanism bequeathed from prehistory.

Clearly, present-day human behavior involves more complex attitudes toward threat than the crudely physical. The modern enemy, whether an aggravating neighbor or the IRS, may arouse primitive instincts, but few would literally run from or fight him. A noise in the night does not startle civilized man from his den as fast as his legs will carry him.

Instead, as heart thumps and blood pressure rises, reason steps in and says, "There's no call for rash action; control yourself." Unfortunately, reason may not impress the autonomic system. Waiting for something to happen, the parasympathetic or calming-down mechanism delays its action. Undischarged anxiety responses remain at readiness. The body is in a state of tension.

There may be a further step. If neither reason nor the autonomic system allays the symptoms of anxiety, the symptoms themselves may become the cause of an "I can't control this" type of panic, "the situation's too much for me. I'm going to faint (. . . have to leave in a hurry . . . make an exhibition of myself, etc.)."

With the parasympathetic branch getting around to allaying the first arousal, its competitor, the sympathetic branch, detects the new panic and steps up its crisis program.

There is now turmoil between the branches, one striving to reduce heart rate and respiration, to return blood to the digestive system and skin surfaces, the other trying to raise blood pressure and respiration and to divert blood to brain and muscles.

The effect is a distressing one, experienced by most people at one time or another. The heart becomes erratic, breathing unsteady, the stomach churns and tightens by turn, the face may become alternately flushed and white, confused muscles tremble, palms sweat and an eccentric supply of blood to the brain can bring giddiness, bewilderment, or actual fainting. Such "anxiety spirals"—in effect, being fearful of the symptoms of one's fears—are not infrequently found along with hypertension. A woman freelance magazine writer recalled:

> The business lunches were my ordeal. An interview can be ended when you've had enough of it, but you can't stop a lunch in the middle without embarrassment. My editors were keen on business lunches. It was not a good time for me because I tended to get headaches in the early afternoon and dreaded that I would get one in the restaurant.
>
> I tried not to think of it, but I would feel myself becoming hot, my hands sticky, temples throbbing. I would think "I must escape,'" but it was too late. I was scarcely conscious of conversation or surroundings. I was going to faint, I would imagine with horror, but somehow I didn't. Iced water helped. I daren't touch alcohol. Instead, I asked for the water and sipped it to clear my head. Then I chose the lighest dish on the menu so that I didn't have to leave too much. I had no appetite. All I wanted was to cut the preliminaries, get the business over and get out of there. People would say how lucky I was, being taken to gourmandize at So-and-So's. I'd have been happier on a bench in the park with a bag of potato chips.

Treatment for hypertension did not banish her anxiety straight away, but it relieved the headaches and she grew in confidence. Today, business lunches hold no fear for her.

TYPES OF ANXIETY

Since an "even keel" is the state most helpful to the treatment of hypertension, anything that can be done to limit anxiety is valuable. The great traumas of existence—grief, pain, dire danger, concern for suffering—are inescapable and are balanced in nature by inspiration and pleasure in life's gift.

For many it is a different type of anxiety, objectively

trivial, even imaginary, that tips the balance and makes control of the fear response desirable. Often, this kind of tension is concealed from the casual eye. Even people as acutely upset as the woman journalist appear self-possessed to their companions through some of their worst moments; others are not aware of their own tensions. Probably they would not agree they felt threatened in any way.

This is because most people think of threats primarily in an objective or "real" sense—a burglar, a house fire, a road accident. And, in civilized society, the possibility of physical threat does not generally worry the average citizen.

Consider driving. The most dangerous maneuver on the road is passing, yet continuous blood pressure recording of motorists has shown that their pressure levels are scarcely more disturbed on accelerating past other vehicles than were they safely at home watching TV. Fit, alert people trust their reflexes to get them out of trouble—even boast of it. "Lucky for that stupid pedestrian I react fast. I avoided him instinctively; lightning reflex."

Indeed, in a real emergency, the automatic response system of the body is a life-saver—sometimes of other lives. But many threats, often those that are most distressing, are not "real."

UNREAL THREAT

What of people terrified by mice or spiders? Or those for whom playing a poor game of golf, or owning an older car than the neighbors, is a threat to confidence and self-esteem? The anxiety engendered in such cases summons the same emergency procedures as does real danger. The same tensions are created but undischarged.

In the case of illogical anxieties, such as the fear of harmless insects, a crossed line somewhere in the learning process of experience has propagated an inappropriate response. Understanding the reason for subjectively assessed threat, or phobia, sometimes helps. Therapy can also often help.

Otherwise, when hypertension is involved, it may simply be best to acknowledge a limitation and give a wide berth to airplanes, crowds, or whatever triggers the anxiety.

Threats to esteem or self-image are another thing. The image a person has of himself, or herself, say psychiatrists, is as sensitive to threat as is the "real" person. In some ways, it is even more vulnerable.

Self-image develops from the accident of birth, of culture, class, and education, gaining character from talents and achievements as life progresses. The fact that it is highly subjective as an assessment does not diminish its importance. Those who live with hypertensives whose opinions they value should remember that to diminish self-image, whether through lack of tact or misplaced jest, is to diminish personality, to lower confidence. Threats to the identity we create for ourselves are deeply upsetting, even destructive. Therefore, people seek to associate with those who reinforce their views of themselves and to avoid those who challenge such views. By the same token, they avoid those who question their *expectations,* for self-image and expectation are inseparable.

To see oneself as a commercial wizard is to expect success; to see oneself as a leader is to expect respect; to see oneself as beautiful is to expect admiration. Challenges to either image or expection raise anxieties that appear absurd in real perspective. Yet nobody, hypertensive or normotensive, is exempt from some such stresses, perhaps in the form of anxiety about what the neighbors think, about how a dinner will turn out, about not having as fashionable a hair-do as a friend. Such things are trivialities that shame intelligence. Intelligence is irrelevant, however. The fact is that people, however sensible they may be, are more likely to experience stress as the result of a scratched motor car or a tactless word from a parent-in-law than they are from world events. To acknowledge the fact is to be prepared.

9

Relaxation

Learning to relax, to respond to anxiety with the opposite of tension, is the key to self-help with high blood pressure. *Re*-learning is perhaps a better way of putting it, for relaxation is a natural condition, as observation of young children makes amply evident. Children can relax as completely as puppies, oblivious of the cares of the world, loose-limbed, flopped-out.

Relaxation is rest, and the body is designed to function on a program of rest and work in which the heart itself spends the larger part of the time at rest. For every heartbeat, its muscle works 0.3 of a second and rests 0.5 of a second.

Everyone needs to relax; it is basic. Tension is needed, too, to get things done. But when tension is created and unused, not only is energy wasted, it becomes increasingly difficult to relax. Lack of relaxation produces stress symptoms that, in turn, evoke more anxiety, more tension.

The first step to breaking the cycle, to banishing tension, is to know the signs. Recognition may be easier when the stress is in others and not ourselves. In some people it is obvious: tapping fingers, hunched posture, knitted brow, narrowed eyes. We know the restless movements, fidgeting, blurted or fumbled words. "A mass of nerves" is the descriptive phrase.

In other cases, concealed by a calm façade—especially where putting people at ease is a professional skill—indications may be elusive except to a trained eye.

The last place many people spot tension is in themselves. Yet it is there in everybody to some extent. Pause a moment between jobs, or when work is over, and make the checks suggested in the following paragraphs.

HANDS

When a person is tense, the fingers tend to curl into a fist, to clasp things tightly, to fidget with small objects—pencil, cigarette lighter, car keys, coins in a pocket. The hands may seek each other, linking fingers, performing "washing" motions, one or both clasping the wrist of the other.

Tenseness can most easily be felt in the hands. Notice how athletes, before competing, let their hands hang loosely, relaxing hands and fingers floppily from the wrist. If there is tenseness, the difference will be obvious on doing this.

ARMS AND SHOULDERS

The upper arms are inclined to press against torso in tension, elbows bending so that lower arms hug the chest or diaphragm. The shoulders are raised toward the ears, giving a hunched effect that will vanish if arms and shoulders are allowed to fall limply and naturally.

HEAD

As the shoulders are lifted, the head comes forward in the stressed position. If the tension is predominantly of fear or anguish, the chin will drop. If it is of anger, the chin will jut out, the head advanced on the neck.

Clenched teeth, a tight jaw, and compressed lips signal tension. People can literally be grinding their teeth and not notice it. The eyes may be screwed up as if in glaring light, or they may be fixed in a glazed stare of preoccupation.

LEGS

Aimless pacing is an obvious indication of tension. Inability to keep still is characteristic of the stressed condition, and anxious people will find excuses to keep moving—"Another cup of coffee?", "I'll just wash-up"—rather than sit restfully. When standing, they will scuffle their feet or repeatedly alter the adjustment of legs and hips.

In a sitting position, their legs are usually crossed in tension, the top foot often flexed rapidly up and down from the ankle while its owner is talking or listening. Or the ankle of one leg may be hooked around the other leg.

BODY

The body tends to stoop when tense and may be pulled up rigidly from time to time, as if on the parade ground, when the curved spine brings discomfort.

Most people have been conscious of one or another of these stress signs at some time.

The amount of tension, of course, varies with the occasion and the temperament of the individual. Intelligent and sensitive people might be expected to develop more tension than the obtuse and insensitive, but all respond to stress with some degree of tension.

Medical tests on a battalion of soldiers withdrawn after two years from active service in World War II showed that most had stress symptoms, blood pressure being so high in almost a third that it amounted to transient hypertension.

In times of deep emotion, pain, or apprehension, people may develop the whole pattern of tension signs simultaneously. Such a response can itself lead to health damage: backaches, ulcers, and breathing problems, among other things. Cardiologists report that simply maintaining a tense hand grip increases blood pressure and pulse rate. In time, changes in the walls of blood vessels may take place.

Although sometimes the fear reflex is needed to support life, the need to thwart the effects of its excessive use is important to persons living in this era of stress.

METHODS OF RELAXATION

It is not a purpose of this book to describe the various techniques that have been evolved to induce relaxation. Instead, we mention one or two to suggest the scope. The techniques are numerous. Some of them are widely practiced, but more are simply the homespun stratagems of individuals.

People with stress symptoms may discover relief by accident. One man, persistently troubled by hypertension-related headaches on the train home from work, found that gazing at the gently rocking pattern of the carriage seat opposite his own induced a mild and sedating trance.

Others find that the calm of an evening stroll, listening to music, or recalling treasured memories dismisses tension. Recreation of all types is usually relaxing, not being associated with competitive intensity.

The surest way to end tension would be to banish stress factors from life, and to some extent at least this may be done by selection of environment—choosing, as far as possible, the home, partner, work, and friends most compatible with contentment and serenity.

Another way would be to gain control over one's autonomic system, and the glands and muscles it commands. Since such muscle interlines blood vessels, blood pressure might be governed this way.

Techniques aimed at restraining the response to anxiety arousal by matching the arousal with conscious thoughts of peace and relaxation may be successful. One method relies on the detection of the fear reflex by an instrument that measures the dampness of the skin as a lead is held. Information is relayed from this *biofeedback* machine by dial or buzzer to enable the subject to synchronize thought with reflex.

A simpler method of conditioning is to make a point of adopting as calm and relaxed an attitude as possible whenever nature's sensory system indicates arousal by that lurch in the stomach, those tensed joints. It is surprising how quickly relaxation can become a habit.

DISASSOCIATION

A practical way to reduce tension and conserve energy, since total relaxation is not convenient at most times, is by what is variously called disassociation or differential relaxation, which is the skill of relaxing part of the body while consciously keeping another part tensed. Too often people use muscle tension all over the body in an activity, instead of merely in those parts needed to achieve their aim. By learning to relax the muscle groups that are not required to be under tension, not only is unnecessary strain spared, but greater confidence can be brought to performance. Dancers and athletes know this; they are trained in the technique. Farm workers, lumberjacks, and others in highly physical jobs instinctively use the technique.

MEDITATION

Doctors have observed an alleviation of hypertension in some people who have tried such contemplative methods of relaxation as Transcendental Meditation. Meditative traditions, including Zen and Sufism, are part of Eastern culture, and perhaps it is no coincidence that hypertension is relatively uncommon among peoples inclined to passive philosophical practices.

The aim of such philosophies as Yoga is to transcend the limitations of bodily systems, ultimately achieving sufficient freedom or grace to effect reunion with the universal spirit. At an elementary level the procedure seeks, like all tension-reducing methods, to neutralize the anxiety reflex through relaxation.

Typically, there is the involvement of some form of hypnotic agent—a lighted candle or bright object—and a focal word or phrase repeated mentally to the exclusion of other thoughts. A passive, unconcerned attitude toward thought and object is cultivated. The man on the train was employing something of the same approach when he allowed his mind to be "taken over" by the rocking pattern of the carriage seat.

QUICK RELAXATION

Meditation, like other advertised techniques that can be learned by book or tutorial, demands disengagement from the normal activities of everyday life for regular and appreciable lengths of time. So does relaxation through sport, vacation, or sheer idleness.

Many therapists recommend a simple form of physiological relaxation that can be used quickly at odd moments of the day—at the office, when traveling, at home—when tension builds up. By physiological relaxation they mean interrupting the spiral of tension by relaxing the parts of the body in which tension is most evident. Variations of the technique exist, but, typically, it goes like this: Sit down, loosen collar and belt if these are tight, let your arms hang loosely and uncross the legs. Let the mind drift from workaday problems to aimless reverie. A kind of mental haze may be achieved by diffusing the focus of vision on a neutral background—bricks, wallpaper—or gazing into space.

The idea is to relax your body part by part, allowing tension to "flop out." Let your hands dangle from the wrists, say the instructors, and flap them limply like a sprinter loosening before a race, so that the limpness travels up the arms. Drop your shoulders and feel the easing in the muscles there and in the neck, too.

Do not, it is advised, let your attention dwell on any one part once it is un-tensed—a matter of a few moments—or concentration will defeat the exercise. Instead, move on. With your head comfortably balanced to look ahead, let your eyelids shut lightly so that your forehead relaxes, and let your jaw sag until your teeth are just parted.

Feel your lips and cheeks relax.

Travel on down the body, which should be upright but not stiff, the breathing light, and let your stomach relax. Do not hold it in, or let tight clothing do so. Let it flop out.

Let your thighs fall open, the knees parting, so that your thigh muscles loosen, the buttocks relax, and the feet tend to roll on the outer sides of sole and heel. The calves of your legs should be "wobbly" and not taut.

Try to enjoy this freedom from tension for several minutes. With practice, the difference between tension and relaxation will become increasingly apparent, and quite small amounts of tension can be located and banished.

People familiar with some such quick and simple method of relaxing find it particularly useful in countering periods of high arousal during the day or working week—getting children to school, business conferences, work inspections, preparing meals, for example.

10

The Family

Hypertension is a family matter. It appears at an age when those concerned are likely to be married with children, it has probably been present in previous generations of the family, and it may or may not occur in some future generation. It will, statistics suggest, be less conspicuous if married couples have children than if they do not, and there is evidence that a family history of high blood pressure may indicate a capacity to tolerate it with fewer problems than encountered by other hypertensives.

During the procreative years, as has been stated, hypertension is somewhat less likely to be a feature of a woman's health than her husband's. Some contraceptive pills raise blood pressure in certain cases, women over forty being less suitable on the whole for oral contraception with estrogen-progesterone preparations. When pressure is increased in this way, usually the variation is small and normality returns after stopping the pill.

High blood pressure in women is often detected during routine prenatal tests. Pregnancy itself may raise blood pressure, possibly owing to an increasing production of renin, or the under-production of substances that normally regulate blood vessels. Doctors are not sure of the reason. They *do* know that effective blood pressure control during pregnancy increases the well-being of mother and unborn baby, and that plenty of rest is a great aid. One or other of the pressure-lowering drugs, maybe methyldopa or a beta blocker, may be prescribed.

Reduction of tension in all members of a family is desirable at any time, for no one member can relax if those closest remain tense. A calm, relaxed spouse is an invaluable asset to the married person with hypertension.

Common sense urges that situations which trigger tension in the home should be minimized. They may be touchy subjects, contacts with neighbors, or encounters with salespersons in a store. Most people have complained of the kind of thing that annoys them:

> "I wish he would stop harping on it, it gets on my nerves."
>
> "Mrs. So-and-So round the corner irritates me, the way she goes on."
>
> "I can't stand that new cashier at the A&P; she makes me furious."

Or there are chores people cannot stand—weeding the garden, washing up after meals, cleaning windows. Not everything that triggers tension can be avoided, but it may well be possible to avoid upsetting topics by mutual agreement. And if one member of the family is made miserable by the prospect of washing up, another sick of gardening, there is no law against breaking habit and changing jobs.

It seems simple—so simple that many people never think of it!

Among the most frequent and potent causes of tension around the home is the cumulative effect of small things that need fixing: a leaky radiator, a wobbly ironingboard, a stained carpet, a loose door handle. It is precisely their triviality, individually, that causes their repair to be put off. But cumulatively, day-in-, day-out, the aggravation they cause builds up until the very sight of the carpet stain, the mere touch of the door handle makes the blood rise. The small effort required to deal with such items is well repaid. Authorities on hypertension emphasize the disproportionate threat minor irritations, often centered on inanimate objects, represent if they are allowed to persist and accumulate.

An understanding of the anxiety syndrome should enable hypertensives and those close to them to recognize trigger factors and deal with them.

If these irritations cannot be removed or avoided, and of course many threats to tranquillity cannot be, then the ability to expel tension by tactical and strategic relaxation is the next defense. It is tactical defense at moments of specific stress, and it is strategic defense when it is a habitual policy.

SLEEP

Sleep, preceded by a soothed state of mind, has been an acknowledged antidote for the stresses of life for countless centuries, and "early to bed" is still among the wisest prescriptions for hypertension.

The best conditions for sleep, experts confirm, are those known to every family dog or cat: a satisfied stomach (though not overfull), somewhere comfortable to lie, and a cozy temperature. A cold bed makes for tension; so does undressing in a chilly room. Masochistic notions about the virtues of discomfort are not appropriate to lowering blood pressure.

Relax, and sleep comes naturally; tense up, it does not. Insomniacs cannot sleep, in many cases, because they are tense with anxiety about not being able to sleep. Their heart accelerates and their blood pressure rises as the fight or run mechanism operates.

If sleep is elusive, as it is for some hypertensives, do not worry, say stress therapists, for when the body is ready to sleep it will. Until then, being awake does not matter a jot. Sit up, if anxiety symptoms become obtrusive, and listen to the radio, read, or watch television. Or try filling the mind with some tranquil mental image: a blue sea creaming gently on a golden beach, a sunny country scene remembered with serenity. Remember the vivid colors, the drowsy warmth. With the eyes lightly closed, belong passively to the scene, letting the body relax in each joint, from fingers, through shoulders to hips and toes.

Hypertensives, among others, may be subject to startling arousals from sleep, their blood racing, heart thumping wildly, chest heaving. A nightmare, something released by sleep from the unconscious mind, has triggered the fear reflex and the body's alarm system has done the rest. Says one physician: "Wake up enough to register a false alarm, then forget it and just wait for the signals to die down. Tune the mind to a benign image, or some pleasurable expection. Relax thoroughly and sleep will return this time undisturbed."

Sexual understanding between spouses is desirable in the avoidance of frustration and anxieties. Hypertensives have no reason to desist from their normal sex lives, and if blood-lowering drugs in any way interfere, they should tell the prescribing doctor.

Some men may encounter a reduction of sexual potency when they are taking certain drugs, in which case the drug may be changed or an adjustment made in the dosing program.

DOMESTIC ROUTINE

Habits may be good or bad, but one way or the other life is built on them. Like all creatures, people stick to familiar ways and, as they age, deviate from them less and less. Although good habits are energy saving and life preserving, bad habits waste energy and put health at risk.

Good habits, ensuring maximum relaxation consistent with achievement, are of special importance to hypertensives. The wisdom of routine, or planned habit, is widely appreciated among those for whom calmness and avoidance of risk is high priority: pilots, seamen, soldiers, firemen, and so on. They are trained in routines that enhance efficiency and confidence. Yet many people eschew routine in their own homes.

They might be surprised to find how far a measure of sensible routine can reduce stress at home and help to stablize the nervous system. The organization of housework as pleasurably and economically as possible, the planning of restful breaks and contrasts to ease monotony, can make for contentment where chaos once reigned. A contented routine and stable blood pressure under treatment for hypertension go hand in hand.

People are too quick sometimes to equate the satisfactions of a quiet domestic regimen with a "stick in the mud" attitude. It does not help the avoidance of tension, investigators agree, to bully or jolly hypertensives out of the leisurely habits they may adopt.

Often, an easy-going, no-hustle manner is the protective coat of the tension-prone person, and while many engage energetically in social activities the preference of others for a quiet life should be respected.

Do not be awed by thoughtless activists. Too often the "She's in a rut, she needs dragging out" type of comment is no more than the verdict of the restless on the well-occupied. "Don't hold back on account of hypertension," advised one doctor, "on the other hand, don't feel obliged to be adventurous."

Many people with high blood pressure fall into the category of those who find it hard to resist demands aimed at their good nature and sensitivity. A polite but firm "No" can be a valuable aid in some circumstances to avoiding stress.

A lot of anxiety, of course, bears little relation to the external world, being largely of a self-centered character—about aging, about appearance, about what others think, about health, about hypertension itself.

Any medical problem is understandably worrying if the limits of concern are not understood. But, as these pages should have made evident, to worry about being hypertensive is self-defeating. To be informed and positive in pursuit of treatment makes sense. Beyond that, trust the natural systems possessed by everyone to take care of things.

Enjoy life; take the advice of those who have lived with hypertension and have achieved high rewards in later years. Stop worrying, they say,

. . . *about aging.* The older a person is, the better the chance of living to a great age with hypertension. Preconception and prejudice based on how people should feel and behave at a particular chronological age has little credibility in fact.

. . . *about what other people think.* On the whole, does it matter? Be yourself, the sages advise; fulfil yourself your own way. Relax. Unaffected people are admired by most, and disapproval from others can be a compliment.

. . . *about appearance.* Countless people persist into maturity with anxieties about minor blemishes of the skin, the tilt of a nose, the size and shape of parts of the anatomy—worries that should have been shed with adolescence. Nobody who has reached the hypertensive-prone period of life should really need telling that courting tension over such things (as if people were prize pigs) is ludicrous.

. . . *about being shy, tongue-tied, undemonstrative, over-demonstrative, unartistic, a stammerer*—the hundred and one things that contribute to the sum of personality. Stop *worrying!* The perfect person would be intolerable. It is the harmless deviations from perfection that provide appeal.

Any anxiety, however ill-founded, can fuel hypertension. Those who live with hypertensive partners can give invaluable help not only by avoiding known trigger factors, but by sowing confidence in areas of self-doubt. Know and sustain a partner's self-image at its weak points.

After all, there are two views of everything. A balding brow may be "distinguished," a spreading waist "voluptuous," a silly taste in clothes "chic," a lack of conversation the mark of the "strong and silent."

One therapist asserts: "A little flattery works wonders for the anxious. Don't despise the old art."

11

Off to Work

Different occupations create different problems in the treatment of high blood pressure. Most of those problems are surmountable with a little thought.

The first thing to ensure is that drugs are not forgotten in the concentration and bustle of the working day, for doctors agree that the commonest cause of difficulty in controlling hypertension is the failure of patients to take their pills regularly. Since the frequency of doses is unlikely to exceed the number of refreshment breaks in a day, and can be timed to accommodate job routines, there is not much excuse for defaulters on grounds of work. Apart from exceptionally heavy manual duties, which may raise difficulties, few jobs cannot be continued quite normally on antihypertensive treatment.

As at home, hypertensives can help themselves by reducing stress. All jobs involve their share of it, and comparative studies do not have much bearing on individuals because temperamental factors play a key role. Until recently, white collar work was held to be more stressful, on the basis of clinical symptoms, than blue collar work. Today, the reverse view is held. However, those who found desk work distressing and switched with subsequent contentment to artisan jobs are legion—as are those who have discovered relief by migrating the other way. So, if options are practical, weigh the pros and cons.

In the type of job where reward is geared to a rate of assembly or packaging, the need to keep pace may create tension, especially in the person who is not dexterous. Or the frustrations of a monotonously repetitive task may build stress.

Other jobs, rich in interest and satisfaction, demand intensity. Work requiring sustained creative or deductive thought imposes much stress, although such work is often thought of as being easy.

All intellectual concentration produces tension, let alone that at professional levels. Watch children, hunched and cramped over schoolbooks, unconsciously chewing their pencils. Watch someone composing a simple letter to a friend and see how the brow furrows, the body tenses. If he or she smokes, watch the stubs as they fill the ashtray.

Whatever the work, heed the warning of tension—the taut muscles, the clamped jaw, the peering eyes. For most hypertensives, mature in age and occupation, change of work is not an answer, but a changed approach to it may be. Once recognized, tenseness, however habitual, can be reversed.

The best insurance against tension at work is variety—variety of thought, posture, movement. "Try," says a leading physiotherapist, "to intersperse sitting periods with walking ones. . . . Tension is often prevented by switching from one task to another and then returning refreshed to the first job." The secretary who has spent an hour or so typing will benefit from, say, five minutes of filing work on her feet. The company executive can help keep tension at bay by breaking his or her concentration periodically—perhaps taking a stroll to a colleague's office instead of using the telephone.

Remember: mental change *and* muscle change are important.

Give the mind a change, especially when problems become intransigent and tension rises as a consequence. Everyone knows that straining for an answer can produce a mental block, whereas the mind often comes up with what is wanted when it is not stressed.

Give the muscles a change, if only by shifting on the office chair, adjusting the body's weight on spine and buttocks.

SEDENTARY OCCUPATION

Work performed on the feet, especially when walking and a variety of other movements are involved, is less inviting of tension than sitting work. Long periods of sitting, combined with concentration, makes conscious relaxation a vital attribute.

Sit comfortably at the correct level for the work at hand, back supported, shoulders loose, legs easy, jaw unclamped. Do not raise blood pressure by holding articles, particularly the telephone, with an unduly tight grip. Many people spend a lot of the working day on the telephone. It is possible to do so in a largely relaxed position, soothing heart and blood pressure as opposed to a series of contortions encourage tension to consolidate.

If the telephone bell startles you, allow your body's automatic alarm response to subside before raising the instrument calmly, reaching for it with the arm only, gripping lightly, not bending the back or hunching forward. Do not tense up when unwanted callers disturb your work, but rather make use of interrupted concentration to relax for a few moments.

According to researchers, opportunities to relax are too seldom taken in another sedentary occupation—driving. Truck drivers, traveling salesmen, and others should make the most of halts at traffic lights and obstacles to shake out tension.

Continuous recording of blood pressure levels has shown that many drivers do exactly the opposite. While driving at speed may scarcely rouse the nervous system, an ostensibly safer situation, such as dawdling in a traffic jam or behind a slow-moving truck often rockets the blood pressure as a result of impatience. Such impatience is largely pointless, since the time involved is rarely vital, but it has heightened tension, speeded the heart rate, and perhaps impaired reasoning.

Few commonplace social situations reveal the unreasoning nature of human responses more vividly than a typical holiday traffic tie up. The sun is shining, there is no hurry to go anywhere, the whole point of the excursion is to relax. Yet what happens when the driver is afforded the perfect chance to sit back and do nothing for a short while? Often, not only a mindless orgy of hornblowing, but even violence offered to blameless fellow-drivers. And to top it, an exhibition of lunatic driving when things roll again. Everyone has seen it—the fight-or-flight response uninhibited, the results as primitive as they are irrational. Hypertensives who drive for a livelihood—or, for that matter, at any time—should be particularly careful to watch for tension in their attitudes.

Are the hands vice-like on the steering wheel? Is the back forward from the seat, neck thrust toward the windshield? Are the eyes screwed up and the teeth clenched? Is the mind obsessed with haste, intolerance of pedestrians, hostility toward other motorists? All people in such a condition are unsafe drivers. The hypertensive are also exacerbating their health problem. They should counter tension by considering both their posture and their mental state. Sit comfortably supported by the seat, hips well back into it, legs relaxed in easy reach of pedals, hands comfortably on the steering wheel with elbows dropped. Stationary moments, such as at traffic lights, should be utilized to rest the faculties.

Relax the body, let the brain work, anticipate. Anticipation reduces the need for snap decisions, arousals of the fear reflex that leave the system revving like the car itself.

On the road, in the office, or in the factory, the relaxed way is the easy way. Do not despise the easy way to life's objectives, for there is no virtue in making tasks unnecessarily difficult just to flatter pride or flaunt capabilities. The master of his craft has learned the simplest way of doing things.

People prone to hypertension are likely to be good at their work, at the prime of their skills and experience. There is no call on them to dash about impressing colleagues or superiors in the fashion of the new hands. Indeed, not only does the experienced professional work better relaxed; others will envy his or her confident efficiency.

Hypertensives fresh to treatment should give thought to working routines that fit the pattern of medication and help to stabilize the inner system. Blood pressure, as has been noted, is likely to be most stable within a familiar schedule, and opportunities to change working habits should be considered carefully.

For some people, adjusting to unaccustomed colleagues and locations proves disturbing; or the responsibilities of promotion may be worrying. Finding the right level in the right vocation, assert hypertensives who have done so, is a big boon.

It may be at the top—hypertension often accompanies drive and high talent. But if not, no increase in money or prestige is likely to compensate for the loss of a congenial routine in exchange for destructive stress.

Finally, bear in mind the following:

1. In most cases high blood pressure is not an illness; the treatment is precautionary. It has been estimated that up to a quarter of the population in Western countries might benefit, were it feasible, from antihypertensive treatment at some time in life.

2. So far as possible, cultivate a livelihood and life-style that do not impose undue anxieties.

3. Interrupt prolonged concentration and labor by rest-breaks or switching tasks, if only momentarily.

4. If help is needed in relaxing, ask the doctor or clinic to advise on the instruction available.

5. Stop smoking, decrease excessive weight, and take exercise.

6. Respect the prescribed medication. Conscientiously undertaken, backed by a modicum of self-help, it will serve well. If adjustment is needed, the doctor will make it in the light of routine check-ups.

7. Understanding the problem is living with heightened insight. Grow with it, mature philosophically, and *relax*. Return to work, to the home, to leisure, a wiser, richer person.

12

A Look Ahead

Hypertension, it was suggested in the first of these pages, has lacked the limelight accorded other health problems. That is changing. In an age of mass information, interest is quickly roused. Modern communications ensure that few people remain oblivious. Already, in some countries, cheap plastic manometers have been produced for sale to the general public, and stores have offered facilities for blood pressure readings as they once invited customers to check their weights.

If misinformation and confusion are to be avoided as a first stage, education must keep pace with curiosity. Then a truly informed public will respond to the care available.

This has been the aim of such projects as the National High Blood Pressure Education Program of the United States' National Heart, Lung and Blood Institute. It takes no crystal ball to foresee increased public familiarity with the problem as an important factor in dealing with hypertension in the future.

Improved doctor–patient cooperation should be one result. Fewer patients, it is hoped, will renege on therapy; more doctors will be inclined to brief patients fully—especially on the kind of drug side-effects which, if unexpected, can be worrying.

Doubtless, the drugs will change. New antihypertensive preparations appear today with such frequency that doctors have a job to keep pace with them. Who can say that the next drug will not supplant the best at present known? Or that research is not already in the process of identifying a correctable causative factor that has so far proved elusive in high blood pressure?

Among safe expectations, it can be predicted that techniques for monitoring blood pressure will much improve, and with them the data bank. Handy and readily available apparatus for the continuous recording of blood pressure in everyday conditions would greatly enhance knowledge of blood pressure behavior in "free" subjects—a big advantage, since periodic monitoring is subject to falsification by transient emotion and other circumstances. "Free" subjects are those being monitored as they go about their daily business.

One authority on hypertension, discussing the possibility of miniaturized personal pressure recorders for hypertensives, has imagined a day when signals from patients would be telemetered to a recording center and printed out by a computer for the doctors. An electronic device might then relay a revised prescription to the patient whose blood pressure required adjustment.

Less fancifully, the installation of cheaply produced computer systems in general practice clinics could make the processing and monitoring of blood pressure data from mass screenings a lot more feasible than it has yet seemed.

Some doctors, however, express doubt that even sophisticated technology would enable them to cope with supervising existing types of treatment at the borderline levels of hypertension if research proved it useful and if society demanded such treatment.

Present knowledge suggests that as much as a third of some populations might then require regular pressure-lowering medication and monitoring. Unsurprisingly, the basic physiological re-education of communities through some form of relaxation program—a concept embracing all kinds of sporting, cultural, and recreational activities—is seen by many as a brighter hope.

In this view, the general quality of life comes into question.

Despite unpromising trends—pressures of over-population, pollution, social disruption of all kinds—a strong body of medical opinion regards environmental reform, in the broadest sense, as the best bet in the long term. Favorable modifications of life-style have been proven attainable where the will exists. People *can* be persuaded to take exercise, lose excess weight, and reduce smoking when the alternatives are put succinctly and objectively. Increases in population *have* reversed in some nations. Environmental interests are being successfully defended against industrial pollution and bad planning.

Success has perhaps been modest, but the full light of necessity has yet to dawn. Among many spurs to enlightenment, hypertension ranks as a strong argument—for well-planned cities, not concrete jungles; for towns ruled by people rather than by motor vehicles; for a way of life that admits the song of a bird above the wail of jet engines and junk "music."

When more is understood of the psychological and environmental causes of hypertension, say some experts, a natural level of relaxation may be obtained that could free the hypertensive forever of drug dependency.

13

Exercise

Although peripheral to the subject of hypertension, exercise is sufficiently important to the prevention of heart and circulatory problems to warrant a special note.

It may be that the hypertensive patient, on diagnosis, already takes part in some form of sport or physical recreation, in which case it is probable (the doctor should be consulted) that it may be continued with benefit so long as pleasure instead of unduly serious competition, is the aim of it. Exercise for the hypertensive should relax as well as make fit.

Exercise can be obtained in many ways consistent with everyday treatment for high blood pressure. Popular pursuits that combine relaxation with healthy exercise and that are suitable at most ages of life include swimming, walking, horseback riding, bowling, and golf. The last two are particularly suited to retired people who may also seek the pleasant diversion of a social atmosphere. Both bowling and golf involve a range of smooth, controlled movements and easy walking. A light-hearted round of golf, covering between three and four miles in congenial surroundings and company, is an excellent way to dismiss stress.

Walking, as a basic exercise, is invaluable to those on an antihypertensive drug regime who find more energetic pastimes tiring. Pace and distance can be adjusted to capability; tolerance of the exertion can be improved by increasing the distance in easy stages.

Indeed, it has been well said that everyone under sixty-five should walk at least a couple of miles a day as routine exercise. Hypertensives often feel at their best in an outdoor environment, with plenty of fresh air and open space. It is not a bad idea, if possible, to walk part of the way to work, or to the shops, instead of taking a bus or car. Allowing plenty of time to find one's own pace, it is possible to experience an indifference to speed and bustle that exhilarates.

City scenery may not compare favorably with rural views, but so far as the heart and circulation are concerned, walking on pavements is as good for the health as walking on country turf. Climbing stairs is also good exercise for heart protection, provided it does not cause pain or undue breathlessness.

All such exertion, taken sensibly and regularly, serves three functions of particular concern to those with a blood pressure problem. First, it provides a cardiac reserve, a measure of power to sustain functioning should a sudden strain be put on the organ, as may happen in a heart attack. Second, it helps to ward off cardiovascular disease. And third, exercise helps prolong bodily mobility in later years, thus facilitating the ability to stay fit.

From middle age onward, immobility is an invitation to declining health. Chairbound periods should be reduced whenever possible in the working day. Both general fitness and the reduction of tension will be served by interrupting desk jobs at frequent intervals to spare time for jobs involving movement. To this end it may be helpful to keep reference books, office equipment, and stationery far enough distant to necessitate a few steps when they are needed. Walking to visit colleagues, instead of interoffice phoning, is also sensible.

Vacations are a good time not only for relieving stress

but for taking exercise. A change of scene refreshes mentally, and the opportunity to leave the car behind and take leisurely walks or join in sporting activities is a boost to health. Unfortunately, many people plan holidays to be physically inactive times.

Too often, the first and last days are spent traveling by road or airplane, cramped and tense, discomfort and delay piling stress on stress. Of course, such travel may be necessary if friends or family live far apart, but it is no help to fitness or to reducing blood pressure. Nor is there much physical benefit in a vacation spent gorging in restaurants, immobile in the sun, or spending more time sitting in a rented car.

That is not to say that those with hypertension should seek exhausting vacations with spartan themes. Some pampering and self-indulgence are good for everyone. *Active, interested,* and *unworried* are key words to consider in any plan.

For those unable to obtain enough exercise through normal activities, or who like to limber up methodically, the kind of "daily dozen" remembered from schooldays or the armed services may be employed. A quarter of an hour a day when fresh and rested will be enough, and no strain should be involved, just easy rhythms.

Simple exercise programs are available in books, on records, or the TV. If the old routines have been forgotten, the following may help to jog the memory.

HEAD AND NECK

Head forward slowly keeping a straight back until chin meets chest; head back slowly, and repeat.

Head turn slowly left, shoulders still, then slowly right, in each case as far as comfortable. And repeat.

ARMS

Arms raise to shoulder height; swing arms forward; swing back again and press gently back. Lower, pause, and repeat.

Arms raise to shoulder height; swing arms above head, pause, return to shoulder height, pause again and lower. Repeat exercise.

One arm at a time, swing the arms in a circular movement a few times.

CHEST AND ABDOMEN

Breathe in, pull shoulders back; breathe out, relaxing shoulders. Repeat, breathing steadily.

Hands on hips, turn trunk to left as far as possible, return to front, pause and repeat to right. Repeat whole exercise accompanying each pause with a deep breath.

Legs comfortably apart, bend from waist reaching for left foot with right hand; return to upright, pause, and repeat reaching for right foot with left hand. Repeat alternatively a few times.

Lying on the back, legs flat on floor, raise shoulders slightly from the ground and lie back again. Repeat increasing the height from ground if possible.

Lying on the back, shoulders to floor, legs straight, raise legs slightly from ground, keep them raised a moment, then lower them. Repeat, increasing height and time raised if possible.

LEGS

Hands on hips, bend knees lowering body, then rise again; pause and repeat.

Legs straight, swing one leg forward until clear of

ground, swing it sideways and backwards and return to ground. Do same with the other leg.

Standing on one leg, raise knee of the other to hip level, point the toes and lower. Do same standing on other leg.

If necessary in the last two exercises, hold a chair to keep balance.

FEET

Standing with feet together, rise on toes, remain on toes a moment then lower. Repeat, also with feet comfortably apart.

Sitting with legs crossed, flex foot upward as far as possible; then the other way, pointing toes down. Repeat a few times with each foot.

Sitting with legs crossed, move foot in circles from the ankle, first one way then the other. Repeat the exercise with the other foot.

It is important to take the exercises gently at first. As muscle tone improves with practice, they will become easier. Five repeats are enough in most cases—ten for the arm exercises and those done lying down. Elderly people and those subject to dizziness should take a doctor's advice about exercise.

14

Diet

Considerations of diet are not central to the modern treatment of hypertension unless obesity is involved, although some doctors recommend a no-salt-added regimen—a reminder of earlier attempts to reduce blood pressure by eliminating salt intake. Among other food factors, the most relevant to the condition is perhaps the attempt by choice of diet to prevent impairment of blood-flow through the arteries. This step, resulting from the cholesterol theory, is still an unsettled issue of medicine.

Cholesterol, a fatty substance in the blood, is found in relatively large quantities in degenerative plaques that may constrict the bore of the arteries. Diets containing high proportions of animal fats, it is thought, produce more cholesterol in the blood than those containing vegetable rather than animal fat. Thus the recommendation is made in some cases, to consume vegetable-based margarines in place of butter fats. Theoretically, this should reduce arterial degeneration and diseases resulting from it. However, practical evidence that this is so is not conclusive.

One experiment based on observing the health of two European groups, one vegetarian and one a normal mixed diet, showed that although the vegetarians were indeed much lower in blood cholesterol, they actually fared worse in terms of disease of the blood vessels. When blood cholesterol is high, the hypertensive patient may be advised to reduce his intake of animal fats, but there are other factors involved—not least the nutritional benefits of such foods—and the doctor will consider them.

Less debatable is the importance of diet for the overweight person with high blood pressure. That excess weight is related to elevated pressures is evident, even in schoolchildren. The percentage of obese children with high blood pressure levels in a sample of American ten- to thirteen-year-olds was more than double that of the nonobese. There is no doubt that high blood pressure in the overweight person can often be treated by weight reduction. In the case of mild hypertension, dieting may be an effective alternative to drug treatment for the obese.

The problem doctors face in prescribing such a method is their inability to ensure that patients in fact lose weight, or, if they lose it, do not put it on again. Although weight-reducing drugs may be helpful, either on their own or prescribed along with antihypertensive drugs, their effect tends to be transient unless supported by dieting and exercise. A survey of more than 800 British doctors who had treated themselves for obesity showed that only 7 per cent had used any drugs. In short, the reduction of blood pressure by weight control demands a high degree of patient self-help.

What is a proper weight? Of course, it varies with individual stature, but most people know when they are too fat. They remember when they were trim and felt their fittest. They can see and feel the difference. Fat that can be pinched in thick folds at the waist, or on the upper arm, is significant, as is a waist that exceeds the chest measurement. A reasonable guide can be obtained by checking with a weight-to-height table, or the doctor will advise those who remain in doubt.

People, as well as horses and other livestock, differ one

from the next in the extent to which they convert food to body weight. Any farmer knows that while one animal is a "good doer," growing fat on the poorest grazing, another will stay thin on rich pasture. There is, it has been demonstrated, a category of fortunate people whose weight is automatically controlled by a self-regulating factor in their metabolism. Regardless of the food they consume, their weight remains unchanged, or little changed. Unfair as it seems, it is no good for the husband or wife of such a person to expect to stay slender on the same meals. Again unfairly, women tend to put on more weight than men. And, in general, they need to diet more severely to take it off.

There is no secret method for losing weight. Weight is gained by the absorption of more calories than the body uses for energy and other needs, and comes wholly from food and drink. Given a consistent energy expenditure, the only way to lose weight is by dieting—that is, by changing one's eating habits.

One method is simply to eat smaller portions of one's normal diet. Many people eat too much, and although adjusting to somewhat less may at first seem difficult, the body will quickly accept moderation as normality. Eating less of the same will reduce weight.

The advantages of a more selective reducing diet are that, by concentrating denial on especially high calorie foods and compensating with lower calorie ones, it may facilitate a sharper loss of weight without a corresponding deprivation of total intake. It should also ensure that vital nutrients do not fall below necessary levels as a result of fasting. This is important because even people with large appetites may actually take less of *some* foods than is good for them. By natural inclination, the sweet-toothed society of the Western world picks a menu overloaded with energy value but understocked with protein, calcium, thiamine, and vitamin C.

Most reducing regimes, whether in the form of calorie counts, special menus, or lists of proscribed foods, work essentially by reducing carbohydrates in the diet. It is the carbohydrates, starch and sugar, that prevent people from burning their reserves of fat.

At the same time, extra proteins may be introduced in the form of fish, lean meat, and dairy products to keep up energy and maintain body cells. Unlike carbohydrates, protein foods assist in the burning of excess fat.

In general terms, then, the weight reducer should avoid the temptations of the confectioner, baker, and pastrycook, and beware at the grocer's. Sugar and some cereal products are foes of the overweight. So is alcohol. Fruits and vegetables are a better bet. Oranges, lemons, grapefruit, tomatoes, and green vegetables are low in carbohydrates, though potatoes and root vegetables are higher in calories. It is the seafood store and the butcher shop that offer the safest havens for most dieters, providing less fattening protein in the form of beef, lamb, game, fowl, and seafood of all kinds.

Such has become the impact of weight watching on the market in modern times that food producers have been eager to cooperate. Sugar-free versions of many bottled and canned products are now offered alongside the sugared stock. Not only is it unnecessary to starve to reduce weight, it is quite possible to indulge, should one wish, in fresh extravagance—instead of chocolates and cake, perhaps a choice cut of meat or a fish delicacy.

The imagination to select and positively relish a reducing diet is important to the overweight hypertensive person. Mentally, it is desirable to avoid regarding weight reduction as a chore or an anxiety. Furthermore, since weight control as a method of lowering blood presure is useless unless sustained, the new diet may become a regular fact of life. Some dieters, back to normal weight, can take more carbohydrates and stay slim. If not, then sugar and starch must be cut again.

Table of Drugs

for the treatment of high blood pressure

Main chemical constituent	*United Kingdom*	*United States and Canada*	*Australia and New Zealand*
Acebutolol Hydrochloride	Sectral	(see chemical name)	Sectral
Alkavervir	Thiaver, Veriloid	Veriloid	Veriloid
Atenolol	Tenormin	(see chemical name)	Tenormin
Bendrofluazide	Aprinox, Berkozide, Centyl, Neo-NaClex	Naturetin	Aprinox, Bristuric
Bethanidine Sulphate	Bethanidine, Esbatal	Bethanid, Esbatal Sulphate, Esbaloid (Can.)	Esbatal
Clonidine Hydrochloride	Catapres	Catapres	Catapres
Debrisoquine Sulphate	Debrisoquine, Declinax	Declinax	Declinax
Deserpidine	Harmonyl	Harmonyl	Harmonyl
Guanethidine Monosulphate	Ismelin, Ismelin-Navidrex K	Esimil	Ismelin
Guanoxan Sulphate	Envacar	Envacar	Envacar

Main chemical constituent	*United Kingdom*	*United States and Canada*	*Australia and New Zealand*
Hydrallazine Hydrochloride	Hydralazine Hydrochloride, Apresoline	Lopress, Apresazide, Apresoline, Dralserp, Dralzine, Ser-Ap-Es, Unipres, Serpasil-Apresoline	Apresoline, Hydralazine
Mecamylamine Hydrochloride	Mecamylamine, Inversine	Inversine	Mevasine, Inversine
Methoserpidine	Decaserpyl, Decaserpyl-Plus	Decaserpyl	Decaserpyl
Methyclothiazide	Enduron, Enduronyl, Enduronyl Forte	Aquatensen (US), Duretic (Can.), Enduron, Enduronyl, Diutensen, Eutron	Enduron
Methyldopa	Aldomet, Co-Caps Methyldopa, Dopamet, Hydromet, Medomet	Aldomet, Aldoclon, Aldoril	Aldomet
Metoprolol Tartrate	Betaloc, Lopresor	Lopressor	Lopresor
Oxprenolol Hydrochloride	Oxprenolol, Trasicor, Trasidrex	Trasicor	Trasicor
Phenobarbitone and Theobromine	Theogardenal, Theominal	—	—
Pindolol	Visken, Viskaldix	Visken	Visken, Prindolol
Prazosin Hydrochloride	Hypovase, Sinetens	Minipress	Minipress, Hypovase, Sinetens

Propranolol Hydrochloride	Inderal	Inderal	Inderal
Rauwolfia alkaloids	Hypercal, Hypertane, Hypertane Forte, Mio-Pressin, Raudixin, Rautrax, Rauwiloid	Rauval, Hyper-Rauw Protium, Rau, Raudixin, Rauja, Raumason, Rauneed, Raupoid, Rauserpa, Rausertina, Rautina, Rawfola, Serfia Serfolia Wolfina, T-Rau, Raufonol, Rautabs (Can.)	Austrawolf, Rautensin, Rawlina, Rauwiloid, Raudixin, Hypothal, Rausan, Serenol, Serpina, Hypertensan, Iserpine
Reserpine	Abicol, Seominal, Serpasil, Serpasil-Esidrex, Tensanyl	Eskaserp, Raurine, Rau-Sed, Reserpoid, Sandril, Serpate, Serfin, Vio-Serpine (US), Alserin, Ebserpine, Neo-Serp, Resercrine, Reserpanca, Serpax, Serpone, Sertina (Can.)	Reserdrex, Ryser, Serpiloid, Tenserp
Sotalol Hydrochloride	Sotacor, Beta-Cardone	Sotacor, Beta-Cardone	Sotacor, Beta-Cardone
Timolol Maleate	Blocadren	—	Blocadren

Some Sources

American Heart Association. *Hypertension—Salt, Hormones & Hypertension.* 1975.

Anderson, Terence W. "Re-examination of Some of the Framingham Blood-Pressure Data." *Lancet*, November 1978.

Buzan, A. *Use Your Head.* London, BBC Publications, 1976.

Dolman, W. "Hypertension: Taking the Blood Pressure Is Just the Beginning." *Modern Medicine*, February 1977.

Edwards, C. R. W. "Aetiology of Hypertension," in *Recent Advances in Cardiology*, vol. 7, ed. J. Hamer. London, Churchill Livingstone, 1977.

Haines, A. P. "Hypertension: Its Appearance and Management in General Practice." *Update*, July 1976.

Hamilton, M. "When to Treat Hypertension." *British Journal of Hospital Medicine*, November 1976.

Hatano, S. et al. (eds.). "Hypertension & Stroke Control In the Community." Proceedings of the WHO Meeting, Tokyo, March 11-13, 1974. World Health Organization.

Hart, Julian Tudor. "The Management of High Blood Pressure in General Practice." *Journal of the Royal College of General Practitioners*, 25, 1975.

Hunt, James C. "Blood Pressure–Regulation & Control." Proceedings of the High Blood Research, American Heart Association, 1972.

"Hypertension." *Update*, July 1977.

Journal Club. "Screening for High Blood Pressure–Is It Worth the Efforts?" *Update*, November 1976.

MacCulloch, Malcolm J. "Psychosomatic Aspects of Hypertension." *General Practitioner*, May 1972.

"Managing Mild Hypertension." Leading article in *British Medical Journal*, 4, 1976.

Marx, Jean L. "Hypertension: A Complex Disease with Complex Causes." *Science*, November 1976.

Mitchell, Laura. *Simple Relaxation.* London, John Murray, 1977.

Parson, R. L. and Fry, J. "Hypertension: Diagnosis and Assessment." *Update*, January 1977.

Parson, R. L. and Fry, J. "Hypertension: Drug Treatment." *Update*, February 1977.

Pentecost, Brian. "Hypertension." *Medicine*, September 1979.

"Report of the Joint National Committee on the Detection, Evaluation and Treatment of High Blood Pressure." *Journal of the American Medical Association*, January 1977.

A Review of Hypertension. London, Roche Products Ltd. 1967.

Sharpe, Robert, and Lewis, David. *The Anxiety Antidote.* London, Souvenir Press, 1979.

Weinstein, Milton, and William Stason. *Hypertension: A Policy Perspective.* Harvard University Press, 1976.

Wright, Beric H. *Executive Ease and Dis-ease.* London, Gower Press, 1975.

Index

S

T

W